Ophthalmology at a Glance

JANE OLVER

DO, FRCS, FRCOphth
Consultant Ophthalmic, Oculoplastic and Orbital Surgeon
Honorary Senior Lecturer in Ophthalmology
Charing Cross Hospital and Imperial College, London
and the Western Eye Hospital, London

LORRAINE CASSIDY

DO, FRCSI, FRCOphth
Consultant Ophthalmologist, Neuro-ophthalmologist and Oculoplastic Surgeon
Professor of Ophthalmology, Trinity College, Dublin
The Royal Victoria Eye and Ear Hospital, Dublin
The Adelaide and Meath Hospital, incorporating the National Childrens' Hospital, Dublin

Blackwell
Science

First published 2005
2 2006

Library of Congress Cataloging-in-Publication Data

Olver, Jane.
    Ophthalmology at a glance / Jane Olver.
        p. ; cm.
    ISBN-13: 978-0-632-06473-1
    ISBN-10: 0-632-06473-0
    1. Ophthalmology—Outlines, syllabi, etc.   2. Ophthalmology—Examinations,
    questions, etc. [DNLM: 1. Eye Diseases—Examination Questions.
    2. Ophthalmology—methods—Examination Questions. WW 18.2 O52o 2005]
    I. Cassidy, Lorraine.   II. Title.

    RE50.O45 2005
    617.7—dc22

                                                                2004011464

ISBN-13: 978-0-632-06473-1
ISBN-10: 0-632-06473-0

A catalogue record for this title is available from the British Library

Set in 9/11.5 Times by SNP Best-set Typesetter Ltd., Hong Kong
Printed and bound in India by Replika Press PVT. Ltd

Commissioning Editor: Fiona Goodgame, Vicki Noyes
Development Editor: Geraldine Jeffers
Production Controller: Kate Charman

For further information on Blackwell Publishing, visit our website:
http://www.blackwellpublishing.com

Contents

Contributors

Jonathan Barnes
BSc FRCOphth
Consultant Ophthalmic Surgeon
Luton & Dunstable Hospital
Lewsey Road
Luton, UK
Chapters 44, 45 and 11

Anne Bolton
Head of Ophthalmic Imaging
Oxford Eye Hospital
Woodstock Road
Oxford, UK
Chapter 41

Susan Downes
MD FRCOphth
Consultant Ophthalmic Surgeon
Oxford Eye Hospital
Woodstock Road
Oxford, UK
Chapters 40, 41, 42 and 43

Veronica Ferguson
FRCS FRCOphth
Consultant Ophthalmic Surgeon
Charing Cross Hospital
London, UK
Chapters 33, 34 and 35

Sanjay Guatoma
Consultant Anaesthetist
St Mary's Hospital NHS Trust

Anthony Kwan
Vitreoretinal Fellow
Moorfields Eye Hospital
City Road
London, UK
Chapters 12, 13 and 14

Jane Leach
The Royal Victoria Eye & Ear Hospital
Adelaide Road
Dublin, Ireland
Chapters 12, 13 and 14

Damien Louis
Staff Ophthalmologist
Melbourne, Australia
Chapter 40

Bernadette McCarry
Teaching Orthoptist
Moorfields Eye Hospital
City Road
London, UK
Chapter 21

Raman Malhotra
Consultant Ophthalmic Surgeon
Corneoplastic Unit
Queen Victoria Hospital
East Grinstead
Sussex, UK
Chapters 41, 42 and 43

Raj Maini
Department of Ophthalmology
Charing Cross Hospital
Fulham Palace Road
London, UK
Chapters 30 and 32

Suzanne Mitchell
Consultant Ophthalmic Surgeon
Chelsea and Westminster Hospital
369 Fulham Road
London, UK
Section 12

Jugnoo Rahi
The Royal Victoria Eye & Ear Hospital
Adelaide Road
Dublin, Ireland

Mandeep S. Sagoo
Fulbright Fellow in Cancer Research
Ocular Oncology Service
Wills Eye Hospital
Philadelphia
PA, USA

Dilani Siriwardena
Consultant Ophthalmic Surgeon
Moorfields Eye Hospital
City Road
London, UK
Chapters 36, 37 & 38

Ursula Vogt
Director, Contact Lens Department
Western Eye Hospital
Marylebone Road
London, UK
Chapters 8 and 9

Preface

This book is intended primarily for medical students and junior doctors preparing for examinations (regardless of whether they are medical or surgical). In addition we hope that general practitioners and non-ophthalmic consultants who care for patients with eye diseases will find this book invaluable in its simplicity and clarity. We have tried to create a balanced, up to date, practical book. Blackwell's have supported our need for extensive colour pictures and diagrams which characterize this 'visual' subject.

Ophthalmology at a Glance took form in London around the time that Lorraine Cassidy was about to go to Dublin to become Professor of Ophthalmology. Slowly we gathered together a team of colleagues and friends who over 2–3 years all pulled together — were cajoled? — into writing this book. As editors we have knitted together our own and their contributing work. We are incredibly grateful to everyone who made this book a reality.

Jane Olver and Lorraine Cassidy
London and Dublin, 2004

Acknowledgements

In particular we want to thank Susie Downes and her team, especially Raman Malhotra and also Damien Louis and Anne Boulton, for several of the medical retinal chapters — retinal imaging, age-related macular degeneration, retinal dystrophies, diabetic retinopathy — all vital subjects. We thank Anthony Kwan for his chapters with wonderful photos on the red eye, eye drops and additional photos of cataract surgery, Siedel positive, etc. We also want to thank Dilani Siriwardena for her enormous contribution to the Glaucoma chapters, similarly Jugnoo Rahi (social and occupatinal aspects), Bernadette MacCarry (orthoptics), Veronica Ferguson (cataract), Raj Maini and Ursula Vogt (corneal and contact lenses), Suzanne Mitchell (HIV), Jonathan Barnes (arterial and venous occlusion) and Mandeep Sagoo (ocular oncology). Others helped at the beginning including Jane Leitch, and towards the end, Roger Armour, Kuki Hundal, Jod Mehta, Arosha Fernandez, Mona Loufti, Nicholas Lee, Karl Southerton, Vickie Lee, Bijan Beigi, Graham Duguid, Eamon Sharkawi, Hugh Nolan and Donal Brosnahan who baled us out with last-minute pictures we couldn't find anywhere. The Medical Illustration Departments at the Charing Cross Hospital and the Royal Victoria Eye and Ear Hospital in Dublin were very supportive. Lastly, Lorraine's nieces had a star role as actresses in the orthoptic department.

1 Introduction: what is ophthalmology?

The medicine and surgery of the eye and its surrounding structures and connections to the brain, in order to maintain clear, pain-free and useful vision with an aesthetic attractive appearance

Normal female appearance with arched high eyebrow

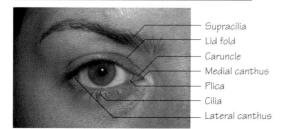

- Supracilia
- Lid fold
- Caruncle
- Medial canthus
- Plica
- Cilia
- Lateral canthus

Normal male eye with straighter lower eyebrow

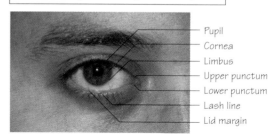

- Pupil
- Cornea
- Limbus
- Upper punctum
- Lower punctum
- Lash line
- Lid margin

Sub-specialties

Paediatric ophthalmology and strabismus

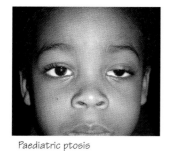

Paediatric ptosis

Oculoplastic, lacrimal and orbital surgery

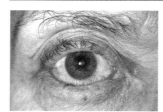

Lower lid entropion

External eye disease

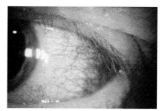

Conjunctivitis

Corneal, refractive and cataract surgery; contact lenses

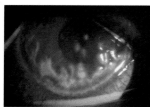
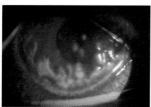

Dendritic ulcer

Glaucoma

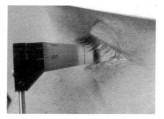

Goldmann tonometry

Vitreo-retinal surgery

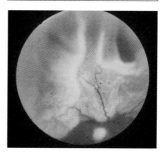

Retinal detachment

Medical retina

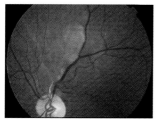

Occluded retinal arteriole

Neuro-ophthalmology

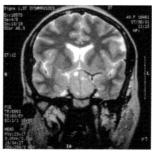

Pituitary tumour

Vision is central to the way we live; our social world, education, mobility and ability to communicate all depend on clear vision. The eyes and the face are important for interpersonal communication – 'the eyes are the window of the soul'. Economically, many occupations are dependent on precise visual requirements

What is ophthalmology?

Ophthalmology is a large subject for a very small area: it is the medical and surgical care of the eye, the adjacent adnexal and periocular area and the visual system. It encompasses the upper and mid face, eyebrows and eyelids, lacrimal system and orbit, as well as the globe and eye muscles, optic nerve and nervous connections all the way back to the visual cortex. Many medical conditions have ocular features as their first presentation, e.g. in diabetes, cardiovascular disease, rheumatology, neurology, endocrinology and oncology. There is overlap with maxillofacial, plastic, otolaryngology and neurosurgery and strong links with dermatology with Mohs' micrographic surgery for excision of periocular skin tumours. There are links with neuroradiology and pathology. It combines medical and surgical skills and uses minimally invasive microsurgery and lasers as well as delicate plastic surgical techniques.

Type of patients

Predominantly the very young and the elderly. Also, middle-aged patients with thyroid eye disease, diabetes or inherited disorders. Ophthalmic trauma affects particularly the young adult. Very few eye patients become ill and die. Most remain ambulatory and are seen as out patients or have day-case surgery.

Team

General practitioners, eye casualty officers, hospital ophthalmologists, medical physicists, optometrists, orthoptists and ophthalmic nurse practitioners, all collaborate in the investigation and management of ophthalmic patients.

Sub-specialties

The eye can be subdivided into several sub-specialty areas. Some ophthalmologists practice general ophthalmology alone; although most have a significant sub-specialty interest. Sub-specialties include:
- Paediatric ophthalmology and strabismus
- Oculoplastic, lacrimal and orbital (including oncology).
- External eye disease including contact lenses.
- Cornea and refractive surgery, cataract.
- Glaucoma.
- Vitreoretinal surgery.
- Medical retina.
- Neuro-ophthalmology.
- Intraocular microsurgery.

How to get into ophthalmology

Good eye–hand coordination helps if you want to do microsurgery and there are ample opportunities for people with good medical skills to practice medical ophthalmology, including neuro-ophthalmology, medical retina and glaucoma, or to conduct ophthalmic research. Examination hurdles are hard. Details of Basic Specialist Training and Higher Specialist Training curricula are obtainable from the Royal Colleges. Getting Part 1 MRCOphth helps you obtain your first Senior House Officer (SHO) post. Do Part 2 and 3 whilst an SHO in **Basic Surgical Training** (BST) (2 years minimum in recognized posts). You have to attend the Royal College of Ophthalmologists' Basic Microsurgical Skills course before you are allowed to do intraocular surgery. A certificate of eligibility is required from one of the Royal Colleges before entering **Higher Surgical Training** (HST) (4.5 years duration), which provides experience in all the sub-specialties. There is exit assessment before being awarded the Fellowship in Ophthalmology (FRCOphth, FRCSEd(Ophth)) and Certificate of Completion of Specialist Training (CCST) necessary to be placed on the Specialist Register. **Advanced Subspecialist Training (ASTO)** towards the end of HST offers further sub-specialty training. Training will be shortened with the introduction of Foundation Training and a subsequent unified training grade.

Membership examination: MRCOphth, MRCSEd

Part 1 Basic sciences. General physiology and pharmacology. Ocular anatomy, physiology, embryology, pharmacology. No clinical experience in ophthalmology needed to sit.

Part 2 (i) Optics and refraction. (ii) Assessment of clinical methods. One year's experience as SHO required. The practical refraction is the hardest part.

Part 3 Clinical ophthalmology including microbiology, histopathology, medical and neurology clinical examination. Eighteen months' experience as SHO required. The medical and neurology parts are the most difficult.

Colleges
- Royal College of Ophthalmologists: www.rcophth.ac.uk
- Royal College of Surgeons of Edinburgh: www.rcsed.ac.uk
- Irish College of Ophthalmologists: www.seeico.com

Education website
- Good basic anatomy and histology: www.lib.berkeley.edu/OPTO/eyeanat.html

Eye associations
- American Academy Ophthalmology: www.aao.org
- American Associated Ophthalmic Plastic and Reconstructive Surgery: www.asoprs.org
- American Association Paediatric Ophthalmology and Strabismus: www.aapos.org
- Association for Research Vision and Ophthalmology: www.arvo.org
- British Oculoplastic Surgery Society: www.bopss.org

Further reading

1 *The Wills Eye Manual. Office and Emergency Room Diagnosis and Treatment of Eye Disease*. Douglas J. Rhee and Mark F. Pyfer.

2 *Clinical Anatomy of the Eye*. Richard S. Snell and Micheal A. Lemp.

3 *Ophthalmology. An Illustrated Text*. M. Batterbury and B. Bowling.

4 *ABC of Eyes*. P.T. Khaw and A.R. Elkington.

5 *Pocket Book of Ophthalmology*. Philip I. Murray and Alistair Fielder.

KEY POINTS
- Ophthalmology is multidisciplinary.
- Interfaces with medicine.
- Involves microsurgery.

2 Medical student aims

Systematic approach

The time spent in ophthalmology is very short so a systematic approach is needed in order to ensure that the necessary skills and topics are covered. Try and cover the items identified in this chapter and refer back to it as a check list.

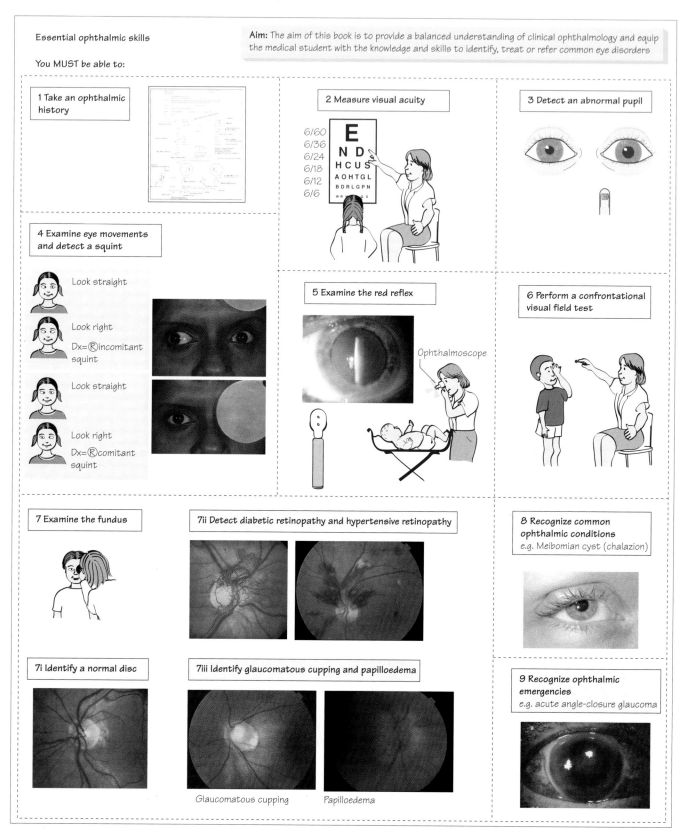

Essential ophthalmic skills

You MUST be able to:

Aim: The aim of this book is to provide a balanced understanding of clinical ophthalmology and equip the medical student with the knowledge and skills to identify, treat or refer common eye disorders

1 Take an ophthalmic history

2 Measure visual acuity

6/60
6/36
6/24
6/18
6/12
6/6

E
N D
H C U S
A O H T G L
B D R L G P N
W R

3 Detect an abnormal pupil

4 Examine eye movements and detect a squint

Look straight

Look right
Dx=Ⓡincomitant squint

Look straight

Look right
Dx=Ⓡcomitant squint

5 Examine the red reflex

Ophthalmoscope

6 Perform a confrontational visual field test

7 Examine the fundus

7ii Detect diabetic retinopathy and hypertensive retinopathy

8 Recognize common ophthalmic conditions
e.g. Meibomian cyst (chalazion)

7i Identify a normal disc

7iii Identify glaucomatous cupping and papilloedema

Glaucomatous cupping

Papilloedema

9 Recognize ophthalmic emergencies
e.g. acute angle-closure glaucoma

Aims

The aim of this book is to provide a balanced understanding of clinical ophthalmology and equip the medical student/physician with the knowledge and skills to identify, treat or refer common eye disorders.

Core knowledge

A basic understanding of:
- ocular physiology and pharmacology;
- neuroanatomy;
- optics.

Medical student objectives

There are **essential ophthalmic skills** such as taking a history, useful **practical skills** such as putting in eye drops, **things to do when you visit the eye department** such as watch a visual field being done and, lastly, **essential clinical topics** such as the red eye.

Essential ophthalmic skills—see figure

1 Take an **ophthalmic history**.

2 Measure **visual acuity** using Snellen and Logmar charts, with and without a pinhole.

3 Detect an abnormal **pupil**, e.g. fixed dilated pupil, Horner's pupil or afferent pupillary defect.

4 Examine the **eye movements** and extraocular muscle function. Detect a **squint** using the cover test. Differentiate between a paralytic and non-paralytic squint.

5 Examine the **red reflex** and recognize leucocoria.

6 Perform a confrontation **visual field test**, and detect a bitemporal hemianopia and homonymous hemianopia.

7 Use a direct ophthalmoscope to: (i) **examine the fundus and identify a normal disc**; (ii) detect **diabetic retinopathy** and **hypertensive retinopathy**; and (iii) detect **papilloedema**, glaucomatous **cupping** of the optic nerve head and a pale disc with **optic atrophy**.

8 Recognize common ophthalmic conditions, e.g. benign eyelid **chalazion** and malignant eyelid **basal cell carcinoma**.

9 Recognize **ophthalmic emergencies**, e.g. acute closed-angle glaucoma, and central retinal artery occlusion.

Additional useful practical skills

You may only do a few of these during your training. Try and do at least points 1–5.

1 Instil eye drops.

2 Evert an eyelid.

3 Examine the eyelids, conjunctiva and cornea with a torch, magnifying aid and slit lamp.

4 Examine cranial nerves including the corneal reflex.

5 Put in or take out a contact lens or eye prosthesis.

6 Detect a lacrimal sac mucocoele.

7 Detect a dendritic ulcer.

8 Remove a foreign body from the conjunctiva and cornea.

9 Irrigate an eye contaminated with a chemical.

10 Assess colour vision.

Things to do when you visit the eye department

1 Attend: (i) a general eye or primary eye clinic, and (ii) a specialist eye clinic.

2 Attend an eye casualty clinic.

3 Observe an orthoptist assessing ocular motility in a child or adult.

4 Observe an automated visual field test being done.

5 Watch a phaco-cataract extraction operation.

6 Watch an eyelid lump being incised or excised, e.g. incision and curettage (I&C) of a chalazion or biopsy of a basal cell carcinoma.

7 See retinal lasering for diabetic retinopathy or maculopathy.

Essential clinical topics

You *must* know about the following topics.

1 Differential diagnosis of a red eye (Chapters 13 and 14).

2 Management of an eye injury (Chapters 15, 16 and 28).

3 Differential diagnosis of visual loss (Chapters 17–19).

4 Orbital cellulitis (Chapter 23).

5 Differential diagnosis of a leucocoria (Chapter 22).

6 Differential diagnosis of a watery eye in childhood (Chapters 22 and 23).

7 Recognition of thyroid eye disease (Chapter 27).

8 Management of diabetic retinopathy (Chapter 43).

KEY POINTS

- Visit the eye department and theatre.
- Know essential clinical topics.
- Gain essential practical skills.

3 Social and occupational aspects of vision

Blindness is a severe form of visual impairment and must be defined. The WHO classification helps:

World Health Organisation (WHO) Classification of Visual Impairment and Blindness		
Category of vision	Level of visual impairment	Visual acuity in better eye with optical correction
Normal vision	Slight if visual acuity <6/7.5 (20/30)	6/18 (20/40) or better
Low vision Low vision	Visual impairment (VI) Severe visual impairment (SVI)	Vision between 6/18 and 6/60 (20/40–20/100) Vision between 6/60 and 3/60 (20/100–20/300)
Blindness	Blind (BL)	Less than 3/60 to no light perception or visual field ″10ϒ around central fixation

Definitions:
BL = Blind
SVI = Severely visually impaired
VI = Visually impaired

Economic impact of reduced vision
A visual acuity of 6/12 (20/30) or worse in the better eye **excludes** entry into the following occupations:

Driving including
taxi drivers

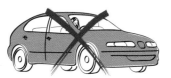

Entry to armed forces

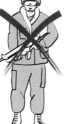

Fire brigade

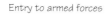

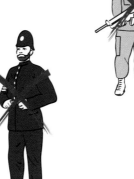

Entry to the police force

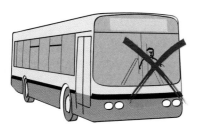

Bus driver

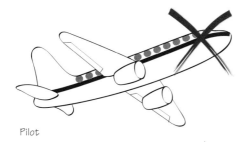

Pilot

DVLA Visual Standards for Driving for ordinary driving licence

N.B. Professional and Vocational licence eyesight regulations are stricter for Large Goods Vehicle (LGV) and Passenger Carrying Vehicle (PCV) licences

- Visual acuity: 'read in good light (with the aid of glasses or contact lenses if worn) a registration mark fixed to a motor vehicle and containing letters and figures 79.4 mm high at a distance of 20.5 m'. This is equivalent to between 6/9 (20/25) and 6/12 (20/30)

- Visual fields: 'a field of vision of at least 120ϒ on the horizontal measured by a Goldman perimeter using a III4e target setting (or automated perimetry equivalent), with no defect in binocular field within 20ϒ of fixation above or below fixation, i.e. total 40ϒ″

A patient can have diplopia in extremes of vision and still be allowed to drive. If in doubt, the patient should contact the DVLA

For LGV and PCV a minimum vision of 3/60 unaided, in each eye, is required, as long as it corrects to 6/9 in the better eye and 6/12 in the worst eye — monocular driving or any field defect is a contraindication

DVLA: www.dvla.gov.uk/drivers/medical/vision-recall.htm

Aims
1 Different needs of developing and industrialized countries.
2 Main causes of blindness in children and adults in industrialized countries.
3 Visual requirements for driving.

Size of the problem
Worldwide
• One adult becomes blind every 5 seconds and one child every minute.
• Approximately 45 million adults and 1.5 million children are currently blind.
• Visual impairment and blindness is very costly from loss of work and managing and supporting them. The global cost of blindness exceeds US$ 167 000 million.
• The WHO 'Vision 2020—the right to sight' is a global initiative for the elimination of avoidable (preventable or treatable) visual impairment throughout the world, by the year 2020.

Developing countries
• Most BL and SVI/VI people live in developing countries.
• Most affected individuals have preventable or treatable conditions, due to infection or malnutrition.
• There is often poor access to treatment, e.g. cataract.

Industrial countries
Most preventable blinding diseases have been eliminated.

United Kingdom / industrialized countries
Children
• Approximately 1 per 1000 children is VI or BL—equivalent to 35–45 children in an average-sized urban health district.
• There may be learning, hearing, speech/language or mobility impairment.
• Major causes of childhood visual disorders include:
  —visual pathway or cerebral visual impairment;
  —inherited retinal dystrophies;
  —congenital cataract and other ocular anomalies such as microphthalmos, and optic nerve hypoplasia and atrophy;
  —retinopathy of prematurity.
• Profound impact on all aspects of the child's development, their family and management by professionals.
• Affects educational, employment and social prospects.
• Although many of the disorders are *untreatable*, affected children may benefit from visual rehabilitation with low-vision aids and specific educational or developmental interventions.

Adults
The incidence and major causes of partial sight or blindness certification in the UK at various ages are given in the table below.

Age in years	Incidence per 100 000 per year	Major causes of VI and BL
16–64	13	Diabetic retinopathy Macular degeneration Hereditary retinal disorders Optic atrophy
65–74	122	Age-related macular degeneration (AMD)
75–84	471	Glaucoma
85 and over	1038	Cataract

A visual acuity of worse than 6/12 in the better eye in adults can be considered 'economic blindness' as it:
• precludes driving;
• prevents entry into certain occupations;
• decreases ability to function in the workplace;
• increases risk of serious morbidity;
• increases social isolation and the risk of psychological problems, including depression;
• decreases overall quality of life and is associated with increased (doubling) overall risk of death.

Services and support in the UK and Ireland (children and adults)
1 National registers of partial sight and blindness. Certification as partially sighted or blind (approximately equivalent to SVI/BL) is voluntary. It is the main mechanism for ensuring access to statutory economic benefits and relevant social services. It provides national data about levels of visual impairment.

TIPS: Certification of partially sighted or blind
1 Both visual acuity and visual field are considered.
2 A patient can be SVI or BL in one eye and even have a prosthetic eye, but if the other eye sees 6/12 with a good visual field, they cannot be registered partially sighted or blind.

---

2 Statement of Educational Needs (SEN). It is a UK legal requirement to assess and regularly review the educational needs of children with SVI in a 'Statement of Educational Needs'. Children registered blind in Ireland are assessed by the visually impaired assessment team (VICAT). The SEN or VICAT report determines the educational placement, support and facilities provided by the government. VI children are educated in mainstream schools with support from an advisory teacher; special visual impairment units integrated within mainstream schools; schools and colleges for the visually impaired; or residential schools for children with special needs.

Useful websites
• Action for Blind People: *www.afbp.org*
• Royal National Institute for the Blind: *www.rnib.org.uk*
• Sense: *www.sense.org.uk*
• National Council for the Blind of Ireland: www.ncbi.ie

KEY POINTS
• Diabetic retinopathy is the commonest cause of blindness in the working age group.
• Age-related macular degeneration accounts for over 50% of blind or partially sighted registrations in Western Europe and the USA.
• Both good visual acuity and field of vision are necessary for driving.

4 Taking the history and recording the findings

Record history and examination: Ophthalmologists use a standard format with accepted abbreviations and notation. The findings for the patient's right eye are recorded on the left hand side of the page and for the left eye on the right side (vice versa for fields)

Name: John Smith
DOB: 23/01/32
Date: 04/05/02

Hospital No. 12345
Age: 70 y/o

PC Slow progressive loss of RVA
   Not improved with new spectacles

HPC Started 3 years ago with glare caused by oncoming car lights when driving at night
   Vision then gradually deteriorated and now can hardly see with R eye

POH Nil   FH Brother with DM

PMH NIDDM x 20 years No hypertension

Meds Daonil 2.5 mg mane Eye drops – nil Allergies – NKA

SH Cigs + 10 per day

O/E

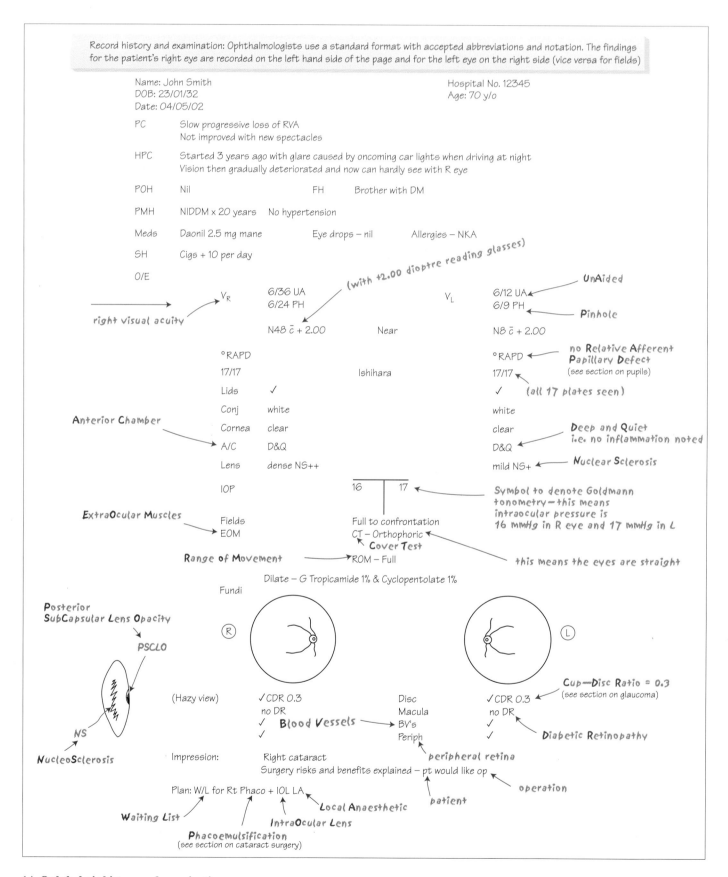

(with +2.00 dioptre reading glasses)

right visual acuity → V_R 6/36 UA V_L 6/12 UA ← UnAided
      6/24 PH   6/9 PH ← Pinhole

    N48 c̄ + 2.00 Near N8 c̄ + 2.00

  °RAPD   °RAPD ← no Relative Afferent Papillary Defect
  17/17   Ishihara 17/17 (see section on pupils)
  Lids ✓   ✓ (all 17 plates seen)
Anterior Chamber Conj white   white
  Cornea clear   clear Deep and Quiet i.e. no inflammation noted
  A/C D&Q   D&Q
  Lens dense NS++ mild NS+ ← Nuclear Sclerosis

  IOP   16 | 17 ← Symbol to denote Goldmann tonometry – this means intraocular pressure is 16 mmHg in R eye and 17 mmHg in L

ExtraOcular Muscles
  Fields Full to confrontation
  EOM CT – Orthophoric ← Cover Test
Range of Movement → ROM – Full this means the eyes are straight

   Dilate – G Tropicamide 1% & Cyclopentolate 1%
  Fundi

Posterior SubCapsular Lens Opacity
 → PSCLO

Ⓡ   Ⓛ

      Cup–Disc Ratio = 0.3 (see section on glaucoma)

NS
NucleoSclerosis

(Hazy view) ✓CDR 0.3 Disc ✓CDR 0.3
    no DR Macula no DR
    ✓ Blood Vessels → BV's ✓
    ✓   Periph ✓ ← Diabetic Retinopathy

Impression: Right cataract   peripheral retina
   Surgery risks and benefits explained – pt would like op ← operation

Plan: W/L for Rt Phaco + IOL LA patient
Waiting List ←   Local Anaesthetic
  Phacoemulsification IntraOcular Lens
  (see section on cataract surgery)

Aims

1 Take a good ophthalmic history.
2 Take a thorough medical history.
3 Examine the eye in a systematic way.
4 Record the eye examination in a standard fashion.

Firstly, always introduce yourself to the patient and explain who you are. It may be useful to record the patients' vision before talking to them, as getting an idea of their visual acuity and which eye is involved, helps you relate to their history better.

Structure of ophthalmic history

Presenting complaint (PC)

The patient may not always volunteer information, and you should ask 'What is the problem with your eyes?' or 'What did you notice wrong with your vision?' or 'Do you know why the optometrist referred you?' Sometimes the patient hasn't noticed anything wrong with their eyes and was referred by the optometrist who noticed an abnormality during a routine eye examination, e.g. early cataract or a pigmented area on the retina.

Establish whether the PC is **acute**, e.g. sudden loss of vision. Ask the patient to be specific about which eye is involved or whether it is both eyes—they may not be sure. Enquire about associated symptoms such as headache, jaw claudication or temporal tenderness which would point to a specific diagnosis such as temporal arteritis.

If the problem is **chronic**, e.g. slowly developing bulgy eye (proptosis), ask the patient when they or their relatives first noticed it—ask them to bring photographs taken a few years earlier for comparison and to help establish how long the problem has been there.

History of the presenting complaint (HPC)

- 'When did the symptom first start?'
- 'Constant or intermittent?'
- 'How many attacks/episodes?'
- 'Any associated features?'
- 'Getting worse, staying the same or improving?'

Family history (FH)

Ask about eye conditions such as squint, glasses and glaucoma, childhood cataract, ocular tumours, any 'eye disease' and medical conditions such as diabetes or hypertension.

Past ocular history (POH)

Ask about previous eye problems, eye surgery or 'lazy eye' (amblyopia).

Allergies

Enquire about drug allergies.

Past medical history (PMH)

Ask about diabetes, hypertension, irregular heart rate, asthma and chronic obstructive airway disease (COAD) as beta-blockers used in drop form for glaucoma should be avoided in these patients.

Other medical conditions including multiple sclerosis, sarcoid, collagen disorders and inflammatory bowel disease may present with ophthalmic problems. Enquire about nasal disease such as sinusitis and hayfever, trauma or surgery.

Medications

- Ask 'Are you taking any tablets/medication?' (you may pick up on diabetes or hypertension which wasn't mentioned in the PMH, especially warfarin or blood-thinning medication).
- Ask 'Have you ever been on eye drops before?' as they may have had previous relevant conjunctivitis.
- Ask in particular about hormone replacement therapy and the contraceptive pill, as both may play a role in the aetiology of retinal vascular occlusive disease. Ask about non-prescription drugs, e.g. aspirin, which can be contraindicated during ophthalmic surgery.

Social history

Does the patient smoke? How many? Smoking may be a causative factor in retinal or optic nerve vascular occlusive disease and is a recognised risk factor in Graves' ophthalmopathy and Leber's optic neuropathy.

Review of systems (ROS)

As relevant.

Systematic ophthalmic examination

Wash your hands first, especially if working in an ophthalmic emergency clinic where patients may have conjunctivitis.

- **Visual acuity** (see Chapter 5). When testing the distance vision, ensure that if the patient has glasses, that they are wearing them! And their reading glasses for near vision tests. Measure each eye separately! Use the pinhole if vision measures 6/9 or less.
- **Visual fields** (see Chapter 6).
- **Colour vision, Amsler chart and pupils** (see Chapter 7).
- **Systematic examination.** Observe the patient's whole person, speech and face as many tips can be picked up—myotonic dystrophy, facial palsy, Graves' ophthalmopathy—as the patient walks in.

TIPS

- Do visual acuity and other function tests such as Ishihara colour, Amsler chart, pupil reactions, visual fields, and eye movements first.
- Examine the eye from the front to the back. Start with the periocular area, lids, external eye, cornea, anterior segment, lens, vitreous, macula, retina and optic nerve head and measure the intraocular pressure.
- Start with the right then the left eye, even if the problem is on the left!
- Only dilate the pupils once you are sure you have established all the above.

KEY POINTS

- Establish if eye problem is acute or chronic.
- Medical history is very important.
- Always measure the visual acuity before dilating the pupils.

5 Visual acuity in adults

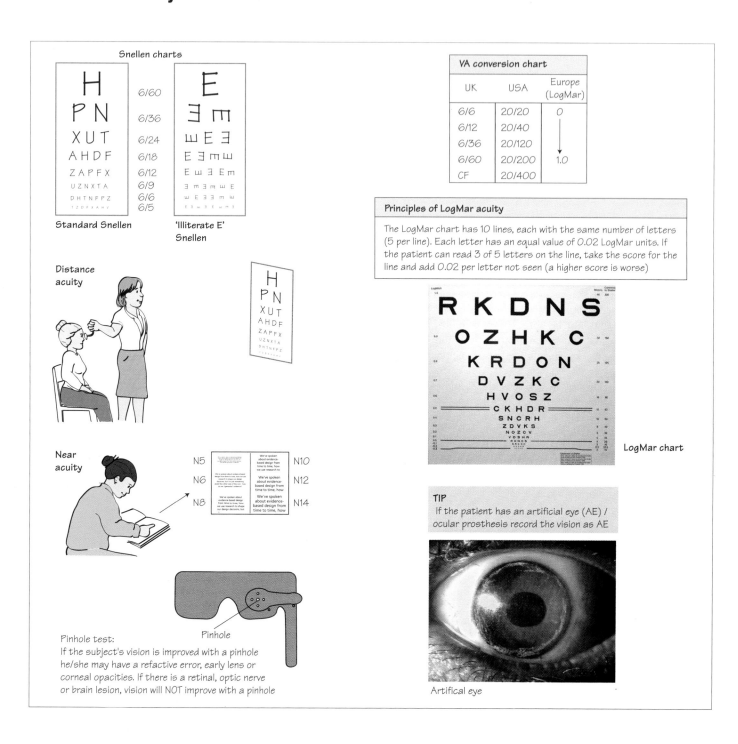

Snellen charts

Standard Snellen
Letters	Value
H	6/60
P N	6/36
X U T	6/24
A H D F	6/18
Z A P F X	6/12
U Z N X T A	6/9
D H T N F P Z	6/6
T Z D F X A H V	6/5

'Illiterate E' Snellen

Distance acuity

Near acuity

N5
N6
N8
N10
N12
N14

Pinhole test:
If the subject's vision is improved with a pinhole he/she may have a refractive error, early lens or corneal opacities. If there is a retinal, optic nerve or brain lesion, vision will NOT improve with a pinhole

VA conversion chart

UK	USA	Europe (LogMar)
6/6	20/20	0
6/12	20/40	
6/36	20/120	
6/60	20/200	1.0
CF	20/400	

Principles of LogMar acuity

The LogMar chart has 10 lines, each with the same number of letters (5 per line). Each letter has an equal value of 0.02 LogMar units. If the patient can read 3 of 5 letters on the line, take the score for the line and add 0.02 per letter not seen (a higher score is worse)

LogMar chart

TIP
If the patient has an artificial eye (AE) / ocular prosthesis record the vision as AE

Artifical eye

Aims
1 Measure distance and near visual acuity.
2 Know why and how to use the pinhole test.

Definitions
• **Visual acuity (VA)**: An objective measure of what the person can see.
• **Pinhole test (PH)**: Simple optical test used to detect the pres-ence of small to moderate refractive errors. (See Chapter 8 for pinhole optics.)

Distance and near vision
VA must be measured, one eye at a time, for both distance and near type, with the patient wearing their best spectacle correction.
• Test the distance VA first.
• Always start with the right eye.

- If the eyelid is droopy (ptosis), use a finger to lift it gently above the visual axis.
- Insert topical anaesthesia if needed, e.g. if with a painful corneal abrasion and blepharospasm.

The methods of vision testing described here can be used in children 6 years and older, but if an adult or an older child has a severe learning disability, then a method of vision testing appropriate to that individual should be used (see Chapter 20).

> **TIP**
> It is important to test both distance and near visual acuity; conditions such as age-related macular degeneration are often disproportionately worse for distance.

Distance vision
- **Snellen acuity**: this is the traditional chart. Snellen vision is measured at 6 m (Europe) or 20 feet (USA).
- **LogMar acuity**: this is increasingly being used for children and patients with poor vision or contrast problems and is useful for research and statistical analysis. The test is done with the patient 4 m from the chart. A LogMar score of 0 is normal, equivalent to 6/6 or 20/20; a score of 1.0 is equivalent to 6/60.

Principles of Snellen acuity
The Snellen chart has letters but there are also versions with the 'illiterate E' and numbers.
- The 6/6 (20/20) line is 'normal' vision—patients can often read the lower lines, 6/5 or 6/4, which is better than normal.
- The number above the line describes the distance the patient is from the Snellen chart; 6/6 (20/20) means the patient is at 6 m (20 feet).
- The number below the line denotes which line is seen, e.g. 6/12 (20/40). At 6 m, the patient reads the fifth line down (the '12' line).
- On the 6/6 (20/20) line each letter is constructed to subtend an angle of 1 minute of arc at a testing distance of 6 m.
- On the 6/18 or 20/60 line each letter subtends an angle of 3 minutes of arc; the 6/60 (20/200) line 10 minutes of arc.
- Each line is constructed in a similar way, so that letters on the 6/18 line subtend an angle of 1 minute of arc if tested at 18 m from the chart, and the 6/60 line at 60 m from the chart.

How to test distance Snellen VA
- Patient sits 6 m from the chart.
- Distance glasses are worn.
- Occlude one eye *completely* using the palm of their hand or an eye occluder.

- Ask the patient to read down the chart as far as possible.
- Repeat for the other eye.
- Use the pinhole (see Chapter 8) if the VA is less than 6/9. If a refractive error is revealed, this patient needs to be assessed for glasses.
- If the VA is worse than 6/60, even when using the pinhole, move the patient 3 m closer to the chart—if the top line is now read record the VA as 3/60.
- If the patient cannot see 3/60, sit them 1 m from the chart. If the chart still cannot be seen, proceed to measure 'counting fingers' vision. Ask how many fingers are held up, and if an accurate response, record as **CF (counts fingers)** and the distance measured.
- If CF cannot be seen, move your hand in front of the patient's eye and if movement is accurately seen, record a VA of **HM (hand movements)**, specifying the distance at which movement was seen.
- If hand movements are not perceived, shine a torch light into the eye from various angles and record whether or not the patient has **PL (perception of light)**, from which direction it is perceived, and the distance at which the torch was held.
- If still no PL, record the vision in that eye as **NPL (no perception of light)**.
- NB, if a patient cannot read use the illiterate E test (see figure). The patient is asked to indicate with his hand which way the E's point.

Near vision
How to test near vision
- Ask patient to wear reading glasses if owned.
- Test each eye separately.
- Patient holds the near test chart at about 0.3 m to read the smallest print that they can comfortably see.
- The smallest print is recorded as N4 or N5 and the print increases in increments to the largest, which is N48.
- Some near reading test types use Jaeger type, which is similar but is recorded as J and the number of the line read.

> **TIP**
> N8 is the most common size print in most books.

KEY POINTS
- Test each eye separately.
- Assess VA before dilating the pupil and before shining a bright light into the eye.
- Test with a pinhole to detect a refractive error.

6 Examination of visual fields

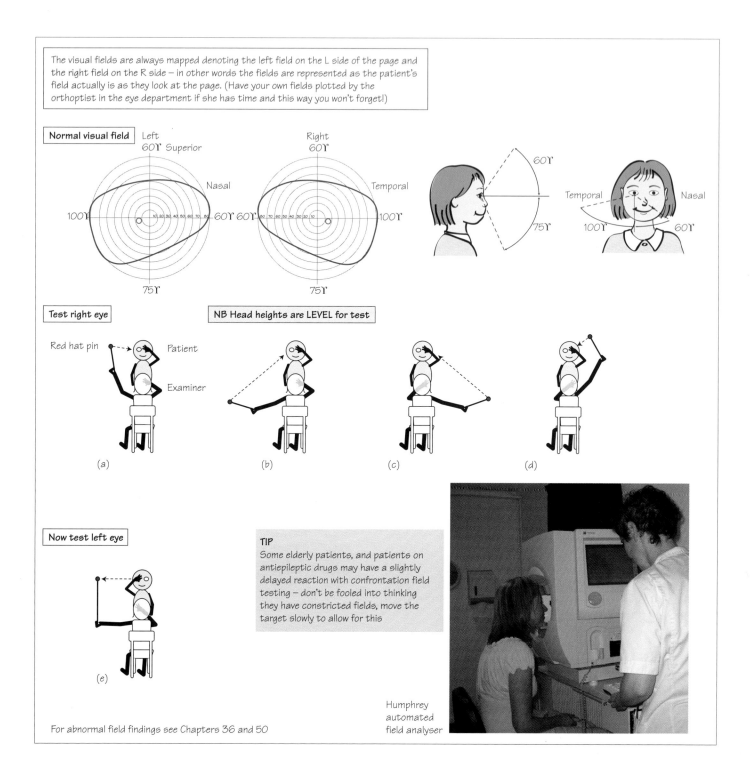

The visual fields are always mapped denoting the left field on the L side of the page and the right field on the R side – in other words the fields are represented as the patient's field actually is as they look at the page. (Have your own fields plotted by the orthoptist in the eye department if she has time and this way you won't forget!)

Normal visual field

Test right eye   NB Head heights are LEVEL for test

(a)   (b)   (c)   (d)

Red hat pin   Patient   Examiner

Now test left eye

(e)

TIP
Some elderly patients, and patients on antiepileptic drugs may have a slightly delayed reaction with confrontation field testing – don't be fooled into thinking they have constricted fields, move the target slowly to allow for this

Humphrey automated field analyser

For abnormal field findings see Chapters 36 and 50

Aim
Examine a visual field by confrontation.

Visual field
The visual field is a map representing the patient's retina, optic nerve and central visual system.

- Test visual fields by **confrontation** for detecting gross abnormalities and neurological problems.
- **Automated static perimetry** is very sensitive and therefore better for detecting more subtle defects such as those seen in early glaucoma (see Chapters 36 and 37).

In your final exam you may be asked to examine the patient's visual fields by confrontation. You should also be aware of other methods of plotting visual fields, in particular the Goldmann, Humphrey and Esterman automated field analysers. The Esterman binocular visual field is useful for driving licence purposes (see Chapter 3).

Normal field of vision

In individuals with normal, healthy visual pathways, a typical map of the visual field is represented pictorially. There is a blind spot temporally in each field—this represents the optic nerve.

> **WARNING**
>
> A person with poor visual acuity (e.g. as a result of cataract) will have a normal visual field if the visual pathways are intact, but will require a large target in order for their fields to be plotted. Don't be fooled into believing that a patient with poor acuity has field loss because you have used a target which is too small—assess visual acuity for near and distance with glasses first.

Examination technique

Necessary equipment for **confrontational field examination**: a red hat pin is best, but a biro with a red cap will do. Red desaturation is an early sign of visual pathway compression.

• Introduce yourself to the patient and ask him if he would mind you performing an examination of his 'side' or peripheral vision.
• Show the patient the target you will be using and ask if he can see it at a distance of 0.5 m.
• If the patient cannot see the target at that distance, ask if he can see where your fingers are, and if so use them as your target as described below.
• If your fingers are not visible, use a pen torch.
• Sit 1 m in front of the patient with your eyes and the patient's eyes at the same level.
• Always examine the right eye first to avoid any confusion.
• Ask the patient to cover his left eye (make sure it is completely occluded), and if this is not possible, cover the eye with an occluder.
• Ask the patient to look at your left eye and not to look for the target. Explain that you are examining 'side' or peripheral vision and instruct the patient to say 'yes' whenever he becomes aware of the target in his peripheral vision (or 'out of the corner of his eye'), making sure that their eye gaze is maintained on your left eye at all times.
• Before you start testing peripheral vision with a small target, ask

the patient if he can see your face clearly, or if any bits appear to be missing. This will pick up any gross field defects (e.g. if there is a left homonymous hemianopia, the right side of your face will be missing or blurred).
• Now present your target equidistant between yourself and the patient, starting outside the field of vision in the superotemporal quadrant of the visual field (a), and bring it slowly in towards the centre, keeping the target equidistant between yourself and the patient at all times.
• Maintain fixation on the patient's right eye and make a mental note of when you first see the target in your peripheral field; compare this with when the patient can first see the target. You should both become aware of the target at the same time if there is no field defect.
• Now repeat in the inferotemporal (b), inferonasal (c) and superonasal quadrants (d).

> **TIP**
>
> An alternative method that can be used if the patient's acuity is too poor to visualize the target is to present 1, 3 or 4 fingers in each quadrant of the visual field while the patient looks straight ahead (avoid 2 fingers so as not to offend). Ask the patient how many digits he can see out of the corner of his eye (vary the number of fingers in each quadrant).

• **Check the blind spot** (if the patient has an obvious homonymous hemianopia, altitudinal field defect, bitemporal hemianopia or grossly constricted fields, there is no need to assess the blind spot). Examine one eye at a time. Ensure stable eye fixation at all times. *Slowly* bringing a small target (hat pin is best here) from the centre, on a straight line towards the temporal periphery (e). Ask the patient to indicate when the top of the hat pin disappears, and when it reappears. Compare with your own blind spot.
• Now examine the left field.

KEY POINTS
• Confrontation visual field tests are good for marked field defects, but are unlikely to detect subtle field changes.
• Goldmann fields are best for neurological defects.
• Automated perimetry is best to detect and monitor glaucomatous field defects.

7 Other visual functions

Left posterior pole – optic nerve transmits all retinal nerve fibres centrally. Macula has dense cones

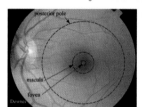

Copyright S Downes

Right posterior pole. There are 6 million cones at the posterior pole. Macula has almost 200000 cones responsible for colour vision
Copyright S Downes

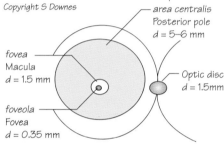

area centralis
Posterior pole
d = 5–6 mm

fovea
Macula
d = 1.5 mm

Optic disc
d = 1.5mm

foveola
Fovea
d = 0.35 mm

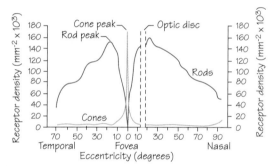

Eccentricity (degrees)

Pupil testing in left optic neuropathy by swinging flashlight test

(a)

Both pupils constricted as a result of direct and consentual light reflex

(b)

Pen moved towards left affected eye

(c)

Relative afferent pupillary defect

Both pupils appear to dilate relative to (a) as less light being interpreted by left affected eye

Colour vision testing is a NEAR VISION TEST - patient must have their reading spectacles on
Do colour vision tests before shining a bright light in the patient's eyes and before dilating their pupils

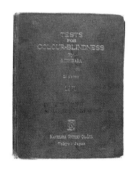

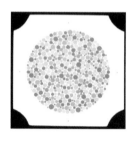

The Amsler chart tests the central 20°

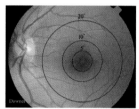

Copyright S Downes

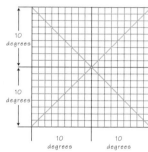

10 degrees

10 degrees

10 degrees   10 degrees

The Amsler chart is a grid given to patients with dry age-related macular degeneration (AMD) to take home and look at regularly. If the lines on the grid become wavy or distorted in a new place this may indicate that the patient has developed a leaky or bleeding subretinal neovascular membrane. This needs urgent assessment to decide suitability for laser treatment

Chart given to patient

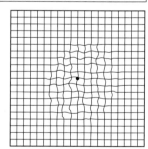

Central distorted lines noted with maculopathy

Aims

1 Assess optic nerve function by testing: (i) colour vision, and (ii) pupil reactions.
2 Assess macular function using Amsler chart.

Colour vision

Colour vision is detected by cones at the macula and is transmitted centrally via the optic nerve. It is a sensitive indicator of optic nerve function and it is vital to assess when there is anterior visual pathway disease. It is also an indicator of central retinal (cone) function.

Optic nerve

• Colour vision is a test of anterior visual pathway function — mainly of the optic nerve.
• In optic neuritis (e.g. may be associated with multiple sclerosis), papilloedema, optic nerve compression from tumour or Graves' ophthalmopathy or any optic neuropathy, visual acuity may be normal and *only colour vision* is *affected*.
• Acquired colour vision defects will be noticed by the patient, and may be asymmetric. NB, a lesion compressing the optic chiasm may cause bilateral colour vision defects, is usually associated with a visual field defect, and may progress.

Macula

• Macular disease due to involvement of the cones, either congenital or acquired, causes a disturbance of colour vision.
• An X-linked anomaly of the retinal cones in males will lead to red–green 'colour anomaly' or confusion. This is the common form of 'colour blindness'.

Clinical assessment

Ishihara

• Assess colour vision using pseudo-isochromatic 'Ishihara plates' — a booklet of plates held at the normal reading distance. Each plate has a series of various sized, colour dots arranged in patterns of hues to represent numbers. Red and green cone function is predominantly tested by this test.
• The numbers are large to aid people with poor vision see them.
• The first plate is a 'test plate', which identifies subjects whose reading skills or acuity levels exclude them from doing the test.
• Ask the patient to read each plate, testing each eye separately to exclude a uniocular problem.
• There are up to 17 plates of numbers; record colour vision as '17/17' if the patient reads all 17 plates, or '5/17' if he could only read five, or 'test plate only' if he could only read the test plate.
• If the patient cannot read ask him to trace the coloured pattern on the illiterate plates with his finger.

Red desaturation

Colour vision can be estimated by the patient looking at a red object (e.g. a red pen) with each eye. If there is an optic nerve or tract lesion on one side the colour looks pink, dull or washed out with that eye. This is 'red desaturation'.

Farnsworth Munswell 100-hue test

This is a sensitive and specific test for congenital colour defects. It covers all cone function, not just red and green.

Amsler chart

This chart (see figure) is a test of macular function and is useful for picking up subtle paracentral scotomas seen in macular disease, e.g. AMD.
• Ask the patient to hold the grid at arm's length and to fixate on the central black dot.
• Test each eye separately.
• They must note whether or not the black lines look distorted (metamorphopsia) or absent (scotoma).
• Ask them to draw in the area of distortion or missing area.

Pupil reactions

The pupil reactions to a **direct torch light (light response)** and to **accommodation (near response)** are important to exclude optic nerve and neurological disease. (See also Chapter 47 for pupil abnormalities.)

> **WARNING**
> If there is gross retinal disease, the direct pupil reactions will also be abnormal due to retinal nerve fibre damage.

1 **Direct light response**: tests gross retinal and optic nerve function.
• Sit opposite patient at arm's length.
• Ask the patient to look past you into the distance (avoids accommodative reaction).
• Shine a pen torch light into one eye and assess pupil constriction — the **direct pupil light response**. The **consensual reflex** is the simultaneous constriction of the other pupil.
• Repeat in other eye.
2 **Swinging flashlight test**: to detect a relative afferent pupil defect (RAPD), which would be a sign of optic nerve damage.
• Swing the light quickly back to the first eye, the patient still looking into the distance — the first pupil should constrict and the second equally constrict.
• Repeat swinging the torch quickly from eye to eye to double check.
• If one pupil dilates instead of constricts, this is an afferent pupil defect indicating a serious retinal or optic nerve problem.
• Always ensure you use the brightest light source available when looking for a RAPD because abnormalities can be subtle.
3 **Accommodation (near response)**: to test for neurological diseases.
• Ask the patient to look from the distance fixation to a small accommodative target brought towards them slowly, up to a distance of about 20 cm.
• Both pupils should constrict equally.

KEY POINTS

• Ishihara plates measure colour vision.
• Amsler grid tests central macular function.
• Swinging flashlight test detects afferent pupil defect.

8 Basic optics and refraction

Emmetropia = Normal eye with no refractive error

Light from sources beyond 5 m is focused by the non-accommodating eye as a sharp but inverted image on the fovea. The brain interprets this as a clear upright image

The pinhole test (PH)

- In emmetropia (more detail in Chapter 9) every point in an object of regard is brought to point focus on the retina and the sum of all the points yields a clear image, i.e. *point-to-point correspondence*

- If there is a refractive error present, a *blur circle* is formed on the retina, which is dependent on the size of their pupil (smaller pupil = smaller blur circle)

- When a pinhole aperture is placed in front of the eye, it acts as an artificial small pupil and the size of the blur circle is abolished/reduced, producing a clearer image

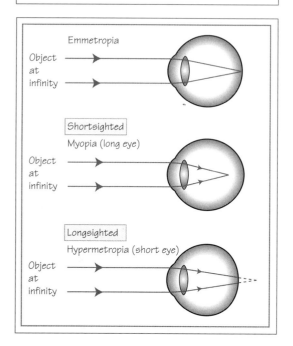

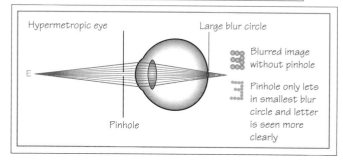

Accommodation

- The ciliary body relaxes and the lens becomes fatter

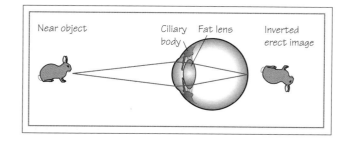

Retinoscopy

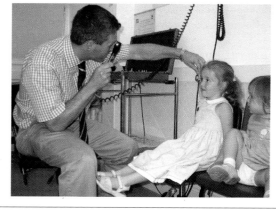

Aims
1 Refractive errors:
- What is longsighted?
- What is shortsighted?
- What is astigmatism?
2 Accommodative changes with age.

This chapter summarizes the basic optics of the eye and defines refraction.

Refraction by the eye
- The ability of the eye to bend light rays.
- Determined by the refractive media (cornea and lens) plus the axial length of the eye.
- It is calculated in dioptres (D) (1D is the power of a convergent lens to focus parallel light at its focal point (f) 1 m behind the lens.)
- The total refractive power of an emmetropic eye (normal

length) is approximately 58D, of which 43D is contributed by the cornea and 15D by the lens, the aqueous and the vitreous.

Refraction techniques
These are techniques for testing the refraction of the eye.

Subjective refraction
The patient distinguishes between the effect of various lenses on the visibility of letters on the Snellen and LogMar charts.

Objective refraction
This includes examination with the ophthalmoscope, the retinoscope or various types of autorefractors.

Retinoscopy
• This technique is particularly useful in testing children under 7 years for glasses.
• In children under 7 years old retinoscopy must be done with cycloplegia (drops inserted to temporarily paralyse the ciliary body and inhibit accommodation; see Chapter 12) in order to obtain an accurate refraction.
• A retinoscope is an instrument used to assess the **objective** refraction of the eye. A bright streak of light is shone through the pupil and is seen as a red reflex reflected from the retina.
• The retinoscope streak is moved gently and the direction of the light reflex from the retina is observed.
• By placing a series of plus or minus lens in front of the patient's eye, the observer can calculate whether the patient is short (myopic) or longsighted (hypermetropic) and measure the amount of astigmatism that needs correcting.

Accommodation
The ability of the eye to focus clearly on an object at any distance, is due to the elasticity of the lens. The **far point** is the furthest distance away at which an object can be seen clearly. In order to see a near object clearly, the ciliary muscle must relax (parasympathetic) enabling the lens to become fatter, and bend (refract) the light rays more, so that they are in focus on the retina. The nearest point, which the eye can see clearly with maximum accommodation in force, is called the **near point**. The distance between these two points is the **range of accommodation**. See presbyopia!

Emmetropia = normal eye with no refractive error
Light from sources beyond 5 m is focused by the non-accommodating eye as a sharp but inverted image on the fovea. The brain interprets this as a clear upright image.

Refractive errors
Correction of refractive errors, see Chapters 8 and 9.
• **Hypermetropia**: longsightedness. Patient can see clearly in the distance but not near.
Optics: The focal point is behind the retina. The converging rays that fall on the retina produce a blurred image.
Cause: The axial length is too short.
Correction: Convex (plus) glasses.
• **Myopia**: shortsightedness. Patient can see clearly close up but their distance vision is blurred.
Optics: The focal point is in front of the retina. Divergent light rays falling on the retina produce a blurred image.
Cause: Most commonly excessive axial length (axial myopia) and rarely due to too great refractive power (e.g. cataract refractive myopia).
Correction: Concave (minus) glasses.
• **Astigmatism**: part of the image in one plane is out of focus due to unequal refraction.
Optics: The parallel incoming rays deform and do not focus at a single point, causing a blurred retinal image.
Cause: Corneal curvature.
Correction: Cylinders (toric lenses), corneal surgery or laser.
• **Presbyopia**: gradual loss of focusing power. The subject is usually over 45 years old and cannot see clearly to read near type. They progressively hold the type further and further away until their arms no longer long enough.
Optics: There is a normal loss of accommodative range with increasing age, due to decline of lens elasticity.
Correction: The reading correction (plus sphere) is added to the distance correction.

KEY POINTS
• The refractive power of the eye is largely due to the cornea and lens.
• Myopic eyes have a long axial length; hypermetropic eyes a short axial length.
• Presbyopia is reading text blurring due to changes in accommodation at around age 45 years.

9 Glasses, contact lenses and low-vision aids

Correction of refractive errors

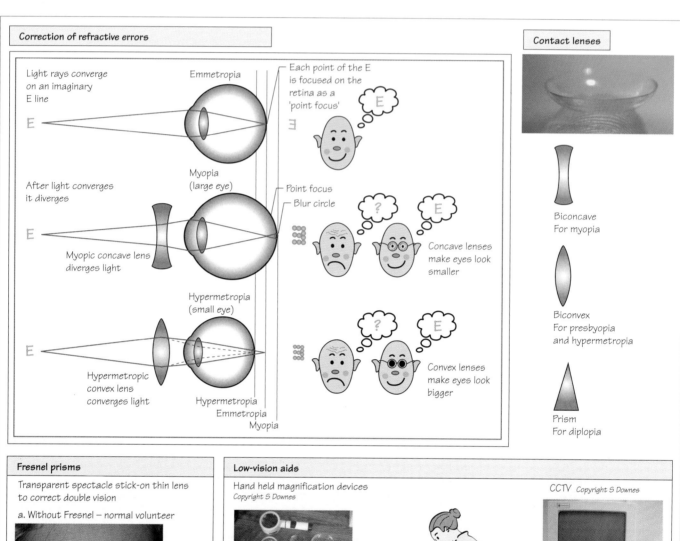

Light rays converge on an imaginary E line

Emmetropia

Each point of the E is focused on the retina as a 'point focus'

After light converges it diverges

Myopia (large eye)

Point focus

Blur circle

Myopic concave lens diverges light

Concave lenses make eyes look smaller

Hypermetropia (small eye)

Convex lenses make eyes look bigger

Hypermetropic convex lens converges light

Hypermetropia
Emmetropia
Myopia

Contact lenses

Biconcave
For myopia

Biconvex
For presbyopia and hypermetropia

Prism
For diplopia

Fresnel prisms

Transparent spectacle stick-on thin lens to correct double vision

a. Without Fresnel – normal volunteer

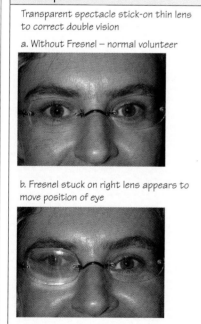

b. Fresnel stuck on right lens appears to move position of eye

Low-vision aids

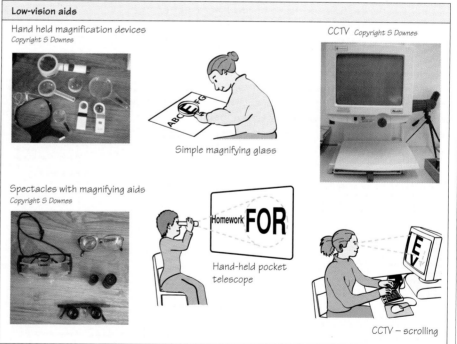

Hand held magnification devices
Copyright S Downes

CCTV *Copyright S Downes*

Simple magnifying glass

Spectacles with magnifying aids
Copyright S Downes

Homework **FOR**

Hand-held pocket telescope

CCTV – scrolling

Aims

1 Correction of refractive errors with glasses and contact lenses.
2 Types of contact lenses.
3 Use of low-vision aids.
For laser refractive surgery, see Chapter 32.

Optical lenses

Spherical lens

This lens has an equal curvature in all meridians.
1 Concave (minus) lens:
  • Used to correct myopia.
  • Refracts light rays making them more divergent.
  • Objects seen through a minus lens look smaller.
2 Convex (plus) lens:
  • Used to correct hypermetropia, presbyopia and aphakia.
  • Refracts light rays to make them more convergent.
  • Objects seen through a plus lens look larger.

Toric (cylinder) lens

• Used to correct astigmatism.
• Shaped like a section through a rugby ball with one meridian more curved than the other (at right angles to each other).

Prisms

• A prism deviates light rays.
• Used to relieve diplopia by redirecting light on to the fovea.
• Fresnel prisms are temporary plastic prisms that are stuck on to the patient's glasses to join diplopia, e.g. sixth cranial nerve palsy.

Contact lenses (CLs)

• CLs are superior in severe refractive errors and give a better quality vision (e.g. correction of aphakia where an intraocular lens has not been placed is best corrected with a convex CL).
• Also used *therapeutically* in corneal disease as bandage CLs or as cosmetic lenses for the scarred cornea. See Chapter 31.

Indications for CLs

• Cosmetic, e.g. avoid glasses in low myopia.
• For sport, e.g. tennis and skiing for wider field.
• Severe refractive errors:
  —high myopia, e.g. ≥6D myopia; a patient with high myopia depends on contact lenses for visual acuity and a wider visual field;
  —aphakic children without an intraocular lens post congenital cataract surgery;
  —irregular astigmatism, e.g. rigid contact lenses for **corneal scarring** and **keratoconus**. In the later stages, surgery (penetrating keratoplasty) may be required (see Chapter 32).

Types of CLs

Hard/rigid CLs
• Polymethylmethacrylate (PMMA).
• Poor oxygen transmission.

Soft CLs
• Hydroxymethylmethacrylate (HMMA).
• Better oxygen permeability but fragile.
• Most common type of contact lens worn for simple refractive errors and as bandage contact lenses.

Disposable soft CLs
• Disposable lens are replaced daily, weekly or monthly.
• Disadvantage: higher infection rate, e.g. acanthamoeba.

Extended wear soft CLs
• Risk of overwear syndrome.
• Complications more common see Chapter 31.

Coloured/tinted CLs (soft or hard/rigid)
Used for prosthetic purpose as hand-painted iris-coloured lenses:
• cover corneal opacities, iris defects or cataracts in blind eyes;
• prevent photophobia and improve vision in aniridia and albinism.

Rigid gas permeable CLs
• Made from a mixture of hard and soft CL materials.
• Transmit oxygen much better than PMMA.
• Good for patients allergic to soft CLs.

Scleral lenses
• A type of hard CL approximately 23 mm diameter that bridge the corneoscleral junction.
• Used for prosthesis purposes and keratoconus.

Low-vision aids

Important in the **visual rehabilitation** of patients with central visual field loss, especially macular degeneration.

Text magnification

Optical magnification with **magnifiers** and **telescopic glasses**:
• Magnifiers increase the image at least ×4 times normal size.
• Telescopic glasses increase the image size at least ×8 times, but cause constriction of the visual field.
• Closed circuit television (CCTV) systems allowing a magnification of 25 times and are beneficial for patients with high degree of vision loss. Expensive!

Page navigation

In patients with macular degeneration, fixation stability is often very poor and they have chaotic reading eye movements using a lot of searching with small saccades. This can be improved by encouraging non-foveal reading.
• Eccentric vision training.
• New methods of presenting text, e.g. electronic scrolled text (i.e. move text to them or serial presentation on a TV screen).
• High tech magnification and image enhancement using a head-mounted CCTV with image processing of contrast enhancement (virtual reality).

KEY POINTS
• Glasses' correction of myopia reduces the size of the image.
• Contact lenses' correction of myopia gives a larger visual field than glasses.
• Fresnel prisms are stuck on to glasses to correct diplopia.

10 External eye and anterior segment

Diagram of external eye

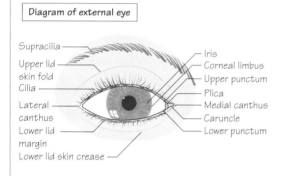

Supracilia
Upper lid skin fold
Cilia
Lateral canthus
Lower lid margin
Lower lid skin crease

Iris
Corneal limbus
Upper punctum
Plica
Medial canthus
Caruncle
Lower punctum

Diagram of anterior segment

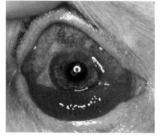

Canal of Schlemm
Posterior chamber
Anterior chamber
Cornea
Anterior chamber angle and trabecular meshwork

Lens
Posterior capsule of lens

Diagram of eyelids

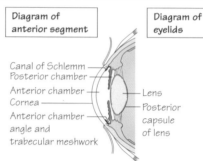

Frontal bone
Pre-aponeurosis fat
Supracilia
Levator aponeurosis
Müller's muscle
Orbicularis muscle
Grey line
Meibomian orifice
Tarsal plate
Capsulopalpebral fascia
Orbital septum
Orbicularis muscle
Maxilla bone

Direct visual assessment with adequate magnification and illumination is required, using a loup and pen torch, direct ophthalmoscope or slit lamp

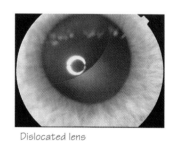

Gross conjunctival chemosis and haemorrhage

Dislocated lens

How to evert the upper eyelid

Place a cotton bud or Minims gently on the upper lid skin crease, hold the central eyelashes and draw them upwards, at the same time pressing gently downwards with the cotton bud/Minims as counter pressure. Ask the patient to look downwards as this makes it more comfortable. Topical anaesthetic drops are recommended to anaesthetize the ocular surface as everting the eyelid can be uncomfortable. See Chapters 12 and 24

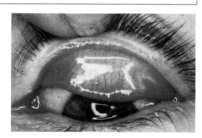

Everted upper eyelid

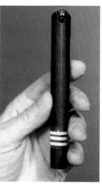

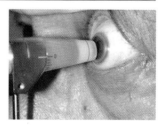

Pinhole
pinhole
Subject's eye
mirror
Observer's eye
Light source

Mini-Armour Ophthalmoscope—a simple pen torch with attached basic optical system. (Courtesy of Roger Armour)

Slit lamp

This provides the best magnification and illumination with a stereoscopic view. The Goldmann tonometer can be attached to it to measure intraocular pressure and a variety of hand-held lenses used with it to view the fundus

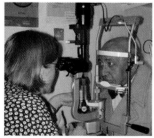

Using the slit lamp
See also Chapter 11

Goldmann tonometry to measure intraocular pressure
See Chapter 37

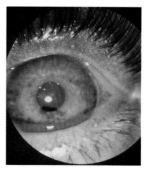

Corneal abrasion staining with fluorescein
See Chapter 16

Aims

1 Anatomy of the external eye and anterior segment.
2 Examination.

Anatomy

The **external eye** includes the eyelids, lashes, lacrimal puncta, caruncle, plica semilunaris, corneal epithelium and conjunctiva.

The **anterior segment** includes the cornea, iris, anterior chamber angle and lens.

Systematic examination

This should be undertaken in the following order.

Lids

• Observe the **upper eyelids** for **symmetry**. If asymmetrical, decide which lid is ptotic (drooping) or whether the other lid is retracted.
• Observe lid position relative to the pupil and cornea.
• A ptotic lid will cover more cornea and may partially or totally obscure the pupil.
• A retracted lid will cover little or no cornea, with the sclera visible above the cornea (upper scleral show).
• Observe the **lower eyelid position** for entropion (lid turning inwards) or ectropion (lid everted outwards).
• Look for evidence of **inflammation**, e.g. erythema, oedema.
• Note any **lid lesions** present.
• Observe the **eyelashes** — any missing? Are they growing in the correct direction or in-growing (trichiasis)?
• When appropriate, **evert the eyelid**.

Conjunctiva

• Use the slit lamp at low (×10) magnification, a pen torch or ophthalmoscope set at +12D held close to the eye or set to zero and held further away.
• **Colour**:
  —Red. Is there injection (i.e. redness?). Does it involve the entire conjunctival surface, a segment of conjunctiva or just the area where the conjunctiva meets the cornea (circumcilliary)?
  —Bluish/purple circumcilliary injection suggests anterior uveitis.
  —In chemical burns, patches of ischaemia appear white, surrounded by severe congestion (see Chapter 15).
  —Yellow. Patients with jaundice may have a yellow tinge to their conjunctiva (icterus).
• **Appearance/texture** of the conjunctiva:
  —Are there tarsal conjunctival follicles or papillae? These are pinkish or fine red velvety lumps.
  —Does the patient have chemosis (conjunctiva has an oedematous jelly-like appearance)?

Cornea

Use the same equipment as when examining the conjunctiva.
• Is the cornea clear, or are there opacities present?
• If there is a corneal irregularity or opacity, instil a drop of fluorescein into the conjunctival sac and note any fluorescein uptake (i.e. staining), which indicates a break in the epithelium. A blue torch light is best.
• Are there abnormal vessels (neovascularization) growing into the cornea? It should be avascular.

Intraocular pressure (IOP)

For eye pressure measurement, see Chapter 37.

Anterior chamber (AC)

Information about the AC is best obtained with the slit lamp. The direct ophthalmoscope (set at +10D) or a pen torch and loup will provide useful but limited information.
• Is the AC quiet, i.e. is the aqueous clear? A slit lamp will show the presence of cells and keratoprecipitates (KPs) (condensation of cells on the inner surface of the cornea).
• Is there a hyphaema (accumulation of blood in the AC)? This may result from trauma, spontaneously ruptured iris new vessels (rubeosis iridis) with a central retinal vein occlusion, longstanding glaucoma, diabetic retinopathy, or in patients with intraocular tumours.

> **WARNING**
> Beware the child with a hyphaema and no history of trauma — think of retinoblastoma or non-accidental injury.

• Is there a hypopyon (accumulation of white blood cells in the AC)? This may be seen in uveitis, infective endophthalmitis, with a corneal abscess, and as a manifestation of leukaemia or lymphoma.

Iris

Use the slit lamp, ophthalmoscope at +8D or the pen torch and loup.
• Notice the colour of each iris. Different colour irides ('iris heterochromia') may be associated with iritis or congenital Horner's syndrome.
• Identify iris lesions: iris melanoma, Lisch nodules in neurofibromatosis or abnormal iris vessels (rubeosis irides), which may signify an underlying ocular tumour, central retinal vein occlusion or diabetes.
• Notice iatrogenic iris changes, e.g. peripheral iridectomy.

Lens

The slit lamp or direct ophthalmoscope is best to examine the lens.
• Use the direct ophthalmoscope set at 0, and stand at arm's length from the patient directing the beam of light to the pupil, to assess the red reflex. Lens opacities are seen as discrepancies in the red reflex.
• Next, move closer the patient at the same time increasing the magnification (usually to +6) until the lens is in focus.
• Detect a dislocated lens with the pupil dilated. It may be caused by trauma, or may indicate an underlying hereditary systemic disorder such as Marfan's syndrome or homocystinuria.

KEY POINTS
• Examine the eye systematically, starting with the eyelids, the external eye and anterior segment.
• The cornea is usually avascular with a shiny smooth surface.
• Cataract is the most common lens disorder.

11 Posterior segment and retina

Posterior pole anatomy

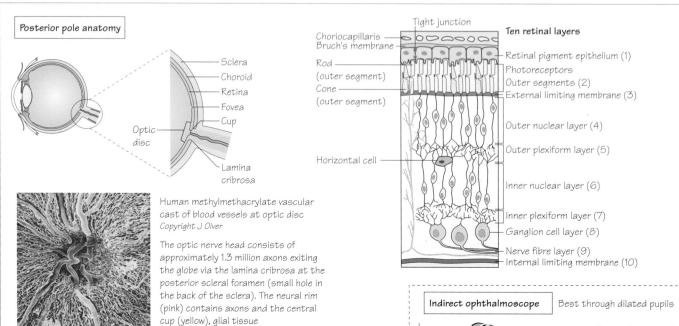

Sclera
Choroid
Retina
Fovea
Cup
Optic disc
Lamina cribrosa

Tight junction
Choriocapillaris
Bruch's membrane
Rod (outer segment)
Cone (outer segment)
Horizontal cell

Ten retinal layers

Retinal pigment epithelium (1)
Photoreceptors
Outer segments (2)
External limiting membrane (3)
Outer nuclear layer (4)
Outer plexiform layer (5)
Inner nuclear layer (6)
Inner plexiform layer (7)
Ganglion cell layer (8)
Nerve fibre layer (9)
Internal limiting membrane (10)

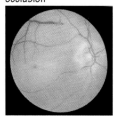

Human methylmethacrylate vascular cast of blood vessels at optic disc
Copyright J Olver

The optic nerve head consists of approximately 1.3 million axons exiting the globe via the lamina cribrosa at the posterior scleral foramen (small hole in the back of the sclera). The neural rim (pink) contains axons and the central cup (yellow), glial tissue

Direct ophthalmoscope

The hand-held ophthalmoscope is commonly used in clinical medicine to view the pupil reactions, red reflex, lens, retina and optic nerve head, even through an undilated pupil. It has a monocular view

Normal optic disc

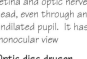

Glaucomatous disc

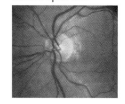

In glaucoma, the raised intraocular pressure causes progressive damage and death of axons, hence they reduce in number, the central glial or empty space enlarges, resulting in an increased cup:disc ratio

Optic disc drusen

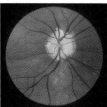

Often an incidental finding but may cause field defects

Central retinal vein occlusion

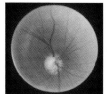

There is a swollen disc with marked venous engorgement and haemorrhages

Central retinal artery occlusion

There is a pale retina, occluded arterioles and a cherry red spot

Drusen (age-related changes) at macula in AMD

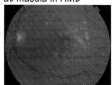

Yellow drusen in Bruch's membrane

Laser at macula

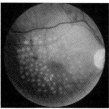

Small regular pale laser burns in retina

Indirect ophthalmoscope

Best through dilated pupils

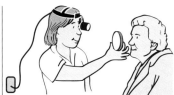

The head-mounted indirect ophthalmoscope is used to view the posterior pole and peripheral retina - binocular view

Useful for detecting retinal tears

Slit lamp

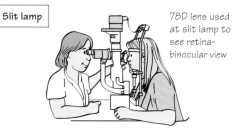

78D lens used at slit lamp to see retina-binocular view

Special lenses are held in front of the patient's eye to view the disc and macula at high magnification — image seen is inverted and horizontally transposed

What you see with each technique

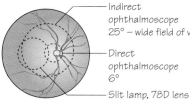

Indirect ophthalmoscope 25° — wide field of vision
Direct ophthalmoscope 6°
Slit lamp, 78D lens

Amount of retina seen with each examining technique

Aims

1 Define the fundus.
2 Understand how to use an ophthalmoscope to examine the fundus.
3 Have observed: (i) the use of an indirect ophthalmoscope; and (ii) slit lamp plus special lenses.

Direct ophthalmoscopy is an essential skill since retinal examination is widely used in general practice and hospital medicine.

Definitions

- **Fundus**: Retina including the macula, blood vessels and optic nerve head.
- **Posterior segment**: Area behind the lens, includes posterior chamber, vitreous, retina, choroid and optic disc.
- **Fundoscopy**: Examination of the fundus.
- **Posterior pole**: Posterior retina including the optic nerve head, macula and retinal blood vessels.
- **Periphery or peripheral fundus**: The retina from the equator out towards the pars plana.

Examination technique

Equipment needed to examine posterior segment:
- **Direct ophthalmoscope**: monocular.
- **Indirect ophthalmoscope**: binocular with 20D lens.
- **Slit lamp biomicroscope** +/− +90D or +78D lens; binocular.

Dilate the pupils

The fundus can be examined with the pupil undilated (best in darkness to ensure maximum pupil size). A better view is achieved if the pupils are dilated.

In adults, Guttae cyclopentolate 1% or tropicamide 0.5% are used, ±guttae phenylephrine 2.5% for greater dilation, especially with brown irides (see Chapter 12).

Do not dilate the pupils

- When pupillary responses are being monitored for neuro-observation.
- when there is a risk of precipitating angle-closure glaucoma (i.e. individuals with shallow anterior angles) (see Chapter 36).

Direct ophthalmoscopy

The light source is focused by a series of minilenses and directed via a mirror into the patient's eye. The observer views the illuminated retina through a sight hole in the mirror. The disc of rotating lenses can be rotated to compensate for both the observer and patient's refractive errors—if both the observer and patient are emmetropic then no lens (zero) is incorporated. The image produced is erect and magnified (×15) with a field of view of 6°.

How to use the direct ophthalmoscope

If you wear glasses or contact lenses for distance keep them on. NB, start with the ophthalmoscope magnification set at 0.
- Ask the patient to look straight ahead.
- Examine the right eye first.

- Stand or sit at arm's length, looking through the ophthalmoscope aperture, directing the light beam towards the patient's right pupil to view their red reflex.
- Move closer to the patient looking at the red reflex until the retinal details become clear, with the patient continually looking over your right shoulder into the distance.
- Examine the optic nerve head/disc.
- Follow the blood vessels out from the disc in their four directions.
- Ask the patient to look up, down, right and left, to examine as much of the equatorial retina as possible.
- Lastly, ask the patient to look straight at the ophthalmoscope light beam to examine the vessel-free macula and fovea.

Assess the optic nerve head/disc.
- Disc margins—should be clearly defined/distinct from the surrounding tissue.
- Disc colour—central cup yellow and pink surrounding rim. If the disc is completely yellow or white, suspect optic atrophy.
- Cup : disc ratio (CDR)—this is the ratio of the size of the central yellow cup to the size of the entire disc. Normally 0.1–0.3 and symmetrical.

Assess the blood vessels.
- Calibre:
  —Are the arteries excessively narrow as in arteriosclerosis?
  —Are the veins tortuous and dilated as in venous occlusion or ocular ischaemia?
- Arteriovenous (AV) nipping, which occurs in hypertension and arteriosclerosis.
- Abnormality, e.g. arteriovenous malformation (AVM), new vessel formation, sheathing.

Assess the retina.
- Colour—retinal colour can vary between races.
- Contour—are there any elevated lesions such as metastases, malignant melanoma or retinoblastoma?

Assess the macula.
- When the patient looks directly onto the light, you should be focused on the macula.
  —Fovea is avascular and there is a sheen from a healthy young fovea.
  —Look for changes in colour and contour in the para-fovea and macula.

Indirect ophthalmoscopy

This binocular head-mounted device with hand-held condensing lenses is used to examine the retina binocularly. It gives a wide field of view at low magnification.

Slit lamp biomicroscope

Is widely used by ophthalmologists for macular and disc examination.

KEY POINTS
- Examine the right eye first.
- Optic nerve cup : disc ratio is normally 0.1–0.3.
- The fovea normally does not have any blood vessels.

12 Use of eye drops

Fluorescein preparations
1 Fluorescein paper strips (Fluorets)
2 Single-dose Fluorescein Minims
3 Combined single-dose fluorescein with local anaesthetic, such as proxymetacaine Minims are useful for measuring intraocular pressure by Goldmann tonometry

TIP
Fluorescein stains soft contact lenses yellow/green therefore these should be removed prior to examination

Eye drops should be applied in the followng way:

FIRST WASH YOUR HANDS
i) Advise the patient to look up to the ceiling and away from the eye drop bottle
ii) Gently pull the lower eyelid down or ask the patient to do so; this will expose the lower fornix
iii) The bottle or Minims is placed directly above the exposed lower fornix, without touching it
iv) Apply the drop.
v) Have a tissue ready to dab the cheek in case of over-spill but not touch the ocular surface

NB After some eyelid operations eye drops are applied **without** pulling the lid down. Instead the patient looks up and the drop is applied to the ocular surface medially

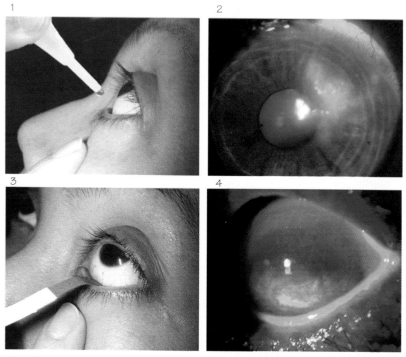

1 Instilling eye drops
2 Fluorescein staining cornea – dendritic ulcer
3 Using a Fluoret to apply fluorescein.
With the lower lid pulled slightly downwards and away from the globe, the strip is gently placed in the conjunctival sac and the fluorescein released
4 Inferior corneal abrasion staining with fluorescein

Iris and ciliary body innervation

Constrictor (sphincter) pupillae
– Parasympathetic
via oculomotor nerve (IIIrd cranial nerve)

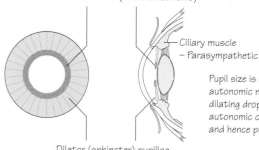

Ciliary muscle
– Parasympathetic

Dilator (sphincter) pupillae
– Sympathetic
via superior cervical ganglion

Pupil size is controlled by the iris and its autonomic nervous innervation. The action of dilating drops is to modulate the effect of the autonomic control of the iris and ciliary body and hence pupil size

Accommodation of the lens (focusing ability) is controlled by the ciliary body which is also innervated by the parasympathetic nervous system and loss of this results in loss of accommodation (cycloplegia) with blurred near vision

DILATING DROPS WARNING !

- Warn patients of the after effects for the next few hours: i) blurred vision – especially for near vision and ii) glare in bright light
- Avoid driving until the effect has worn off
- Risk of precipitating an attack of acute angle closure glaucoma in patients with a narrow iridocorneal angle: the patient must see an ophthalmologist urgently if symptoms of blurred vision persist and a halo effect around a light source occurs

Aims
1 Understand the indications for fluorescein, and the use of common dilating and anaesthetic drops.
2 Know how to instill eye drops correctly.
3 Be aware of the risks of dilating drops.

Definitions
Mydriatic: Drop that causes mydriasis (pupil dilation).
Miotic: Drop that causes miosis (pupil contriction).
Cycloplegia: Loss of accommodation caused by blocking the parasympathetic innervation to the ciliary body.

Drops for ocular surface examination
Fluorescein
Fluorescein is an orange-brown crystalline substance and belongs to the triphenylmethane dyes. It is available as Minims drops or dried onto paper (Fluoret). It adopts its characteristic yellow-green colour after dilution. Use a cobalt blue light from a slit lamp or direct ophthalmoscope to see the typical green-yellow fluorescence.
- Absorbtion spectrum: 465 and 490 nm (blue end).
- Emission spectrum: 520 and 530 nm (green-yellow region).

Fluorescein is water-soluble and does not stain corneal epithelium (hydrophobic). It does stain Bowman's membrane and stroma in an epithelial defect, e.g. dendritic ulcer.

Rose Bengal
Rose Bengal is a red soluble dye and belongs to the group of fluorine dyes. It is available as a 1% Minims preparation. It stains wherever there is insufficient protection of the preocular tear film:
- Decreased tear components, e.g. keratoconjunctivitis sicca.
- Abnormal surface epithelial cells, e.g. degenerating or dead cells.
- Mucous strands.

After staining, cells loose their vitality. Rose Bengal should be used very sparingly, as it causes stinging due to its acid properties. It is advisable to instil topical anaesthetic prior to its use and warn the patient about discomfort.

Common dilating drops for fundal examination
In order to examine the fundus adequately, the pupil needs to be dilated.

Tropicamide 1%
This is a synthetic analogue of atropine. It reduces the parasympathetic innervation to both the sphincter pupillae and the ciliary body, resulting in a marked mydriatic action and weak cycloplegic action. It is used alone or in combination with phenylephrine for better dilation.
- Maximum effect after 20–30 min.
- Effect wears off after at least 6 h.

Phenylephrine 2.5%
This is a synthetic compound and is biochemically closely related to adrenaline; it acts as a potent sympathomimetic. It stimulates dilator pupillae and causes mydriasis. However, the dilator pupillae is a weaker muscle than the sphincter pupillae, hence the mydriatic effect of phenylephrine is less than tropicamide. It is used in combination with tropicamide or cyclopentolate. Useful to help maximize dilation in dark brown irides.
- Maximum effect after 30 min.
- Effect wears off after 5 h.
- Phenylephrine 10% is rarely used due to systemic side effects.

Cyclopentolate 0.5% and 1%
This is a synthetic substance similar to atropine and has the advantage of being short acting and having a greater cycloplegic effect than tropicamide. It is commonly used in refraction in children to abolish accommodation.
- Mydriasis and cycloplegia within 20–30 min.
- Maximum cycloplegic effect lasts 45–60 min.
- Effect wears off after 24 h.

Side effects: risk of allergic reaction and raised intraocular pressure. In a baby <3 months old, cyclopentolate 0.5% should be used. Hypersensitivity is less common than with atropine. Rare side effects: visual hallucinations, disorientation and ataxia.

In patients with darkly pigmented irides, the cyclopentolate effect may be insufficient for full cycloplegia, therefore use **atropine 1% drops**. NB, atropine has a longer acting period and higher risk of side effects.

Topical anaesthetic drops
Topical anaesthesia is used for:
- ocular examination (tonometry and gonioscopy);
- contact lens fitting;
- to alleviate pain due to injury and to facilitate thorough examination, e.g. for a foreign body, abrasion or ulcer;
- in children prior to instillation of often stingy eye drops.

They must be used sparingly and in short courses as they potentially mask the severity of pain if the injury worsens. Prolonged use is epithelial toxic.

Mode of action: prevent generation and conduction of nerve impulses—mostly belong to amine group of compounds.

Anaesthetic drops are obtainable in Minims without preservatives or in bottles with preservatives.

Oxybuprocaine 0.4% (Benoxinate)
Well absorbed with onset of action within 60 s. One drop lasts approximately 15 min.

Tetracaine 0.5% and 1.0% (Amethocaine)
Onset within 60 s and effect lasts 20 min. Contact dermatitis has been reported.

Proxymetacaine 0.5% (Ophthaine)
Onset 30 s, lasts 15 min. It is less stingy than the above anaesthetic drops, therefore useful in children. Also available as a combination with fluorescein in Minims, and useful for Goldmann contact tonometry.

KEY POINTS
- Fluorescein needs a blue light to visualize its yellow colour.
- Rose Bengal stains devitalized cells but should be used sparingly as it stings.
- Tropicamide and cyclopentolate dilating drops also cause cycloplegia (blurring of near vision).
- Proxymetacaine is the only topical anaesthetic that does not sting.

13 The red eye

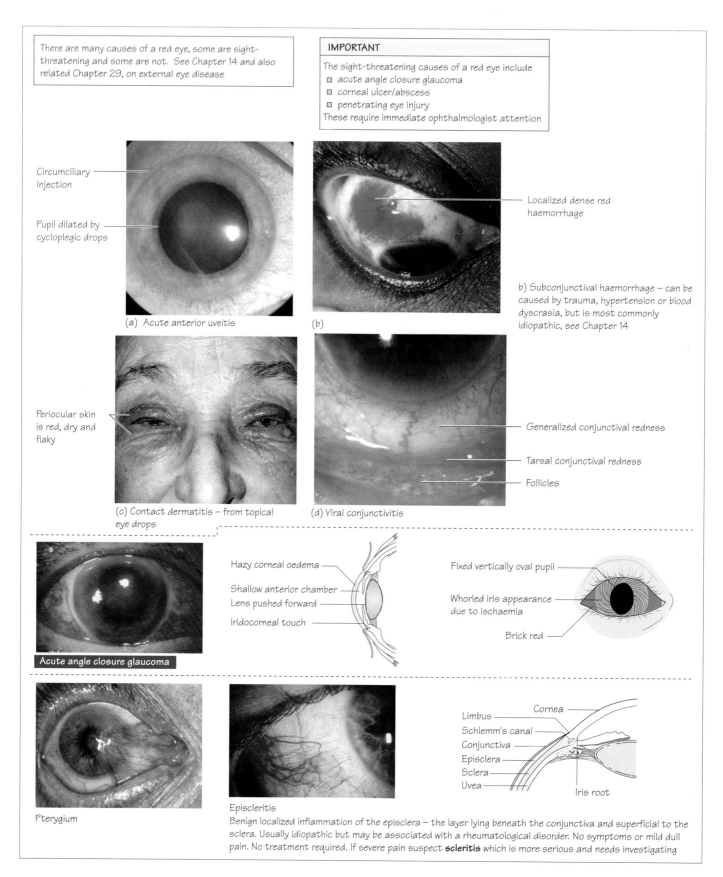

There are many causes of a red eye, some are sight-threatening and some are not. See Chapter 14 and also related Chapter 29, on external eye disease

IMPORTANT

The sight-threatening causes of a red eye include
- acute angle closure glaucoma
- corneal ulcer/abscess
- penetrating eye injury

These require immediate ophthalmologist attention

Circumciliary injection

Pupil dilated by cycloplegic drops

(a) Acute anterior uveitis

Localized dense red haemorrhage

(b)

b) Subconjunctival haemorrhage – can be caused by trauma, hypertension or blood dyscrasia, but is most commonly idiopathic, see Chapter 14

Periocular skin is red, dry and flaky

(c) Contact dermatitis – from topical eye drops

Generalized conjunctival redness

Tarsal conjunctival redness

Follicles

(d) Viral conjunctivitis

Acute angle closure glaucoma

Hazy corneal oedema

Shallow anterior chamber

Lens pushed forward

Iridocorneal touch

Fixed vertically oval pupil

Whorled iris appearance due to ischaemia

Brick red

Pterygium

Episcleritis

Benign localized inflammation of the episclera – the layer lying beneath the conjunctiva and superficial to the sclera. Usually idiopathic but may be associated with a rheumatological disorder. No symptoms or mild dull pain. No treatment required. If severe pain suspect **scleritis** which is more serious and needs investigating

Limbus
Cornea
Schlemm's canal
Conjunctiva
Episclera
Sclera
Uvea
Iris root

Aims of Chapters 13 and 14

1 Identify the four most common causes of a red eye.
2 Understand how the distribution of redness helps make the diagnosis.
3 Recognize sight-threatening red eye.

> Red eye is the presenting symptom of a variety of ocular problems. The most important symptoms are visual loss and pain, which suggest serious conditions.

Infective conjunctivitis

Symptoms
- Red eye.
- Discomfort or itch.
- Discharge (watery or purulent).
- Crusting of lid margins
- General flu-like symptoms in viral cases.
- History of contact with people with red eyes.

Signs
- Generalized redness of conjunctiva and especially the tarsal conjunctiva (posterior surface of the lids).
- Cervical lymphadenopathy in viral cases.

Management
- Hygiene advice, e.g. avoid sharing towels.
- In purulent cases, swab for C&S (culture and sensitivity).
- Prescribe topical antibiotics, e.g. chloramphenicol hourly for 1 day then qds for 1 week or fusidic acid bd for 1 week.

Special consideration
- **Chlamydial conjunctivitis** should be suspected in adults with bilateral chronic conjunctivitis with or without a history of venereal disease. Corneal scarring is a risk, and referral to ophthalmologist is recommended.
- **Ophthalmia neonatorum** is conjunctivitis in newborns less than 1 month old. It is a reportable disease and immediate ophthalmic referral is recommended. In cases of gonococcal infection there is a danger of visual loss due to corneal involvement.

Corneal ulcer/keratitis/abscess

Symptoms
- Painful red eye in a patient who may give a history of wearing contact lens, foreign material injuring the eye, facial cold sores or similar previous episodes.
- Photophobia.
- Purulent discharge is seen in bacterial cases.

Signs
- May have decreased visual acuity depending on the location of the ulcer (keratitis).
- Pus in fornices in bacterial cases.
- Decreased corneal sensation with dendritic corneal ulcer.
- Fluorescein staining reveals area of epithelial defect under cobalt blue light.

Management
- Immediate ophthalmological opinion plus corneal scrape as risk of perforation and permanent central corneal scar.

- Antiviral ointment (e.g. Aciclovir five times per day) is used for herpes simplex virus (HSV) dendritic ulcer.

> **WARNING**
> ***Never*** give steroids for HSV dendritic ulcer—they exacerbate the condition (steroids can only be used by an ophthalmologist in combination with Aciclovir once the epithelium has healed to prevent scarring)

- Intensive antibiotic drops are required for bacterial ulcer (e.g. ofloxacin hourly).
- Acanthoamoeba corneal ulcer can be seen in soft contact lens wearers—beware as pain is disproportionately greater than appearance of the eye.

Uveitis

Inflammation of the uveal tract: iris, ciliary body and choroid.

Symptoms
- Painful and red.
- Photophobic eye with or without a history of autoimmune disease (e.g. ankylosing spondylitis, inflammatory bowel disease, sarcoidosis) or infection (e.g. toxoplasmosis).
- Blurred vision or floaters.

Signs
- Ciliary/circumcorneal injection (engorgement of episcleral vessels around the iris root).
- Reduced visual acuity.
- ±Sluggish or irregular pupil due to reflex sphinter spasm or inflammatory adhesions of iris to the anterior lens surface (posterior synechiae).
- Iris details may be hazy due to inflammatory cells in the aqueous.
- Tiny round opacities may be visible on the inferior posterior corneal surface keratitic precipitates (inflammatory cells on the corneal endothelium).
- Raised intraocular pressure because of inflammation or adhesion of iris and cornea (anterior synechia), which hinders drainage of the aqueous.
- Cataract is seen in recurrent or chronic uveitis.

Management
- Refer the patient to an ophthalmologist for further investigation and management. For uveitis the treatment is a reducing regimen of topical steroid (e.g. dexamethasone 0.1%) to reduce the inflammation and a cycloplegic and dilating drop (e.g. cyclopentolate 1%) for pain relief and prevention of synechiae formation.

Acute angle-closure glaucoma

A sudden rise in intraocular pressure due to closed iridocorneal drainage angle. (See Chapters 36 and 38.)

> **WARNING**
> If diagnosis is delayed, vision can be lost. *Urgent* treatment is required.

KEY POINTS
- A subconjunctival haemorrhage is usually idiopathic.
- Common causes of red eye are conjunctivitis, keratitis, uveitis and acute angle-closure glaucoma.
- Untreated angle-closure glaucoma blinds.

14 More on the red eye

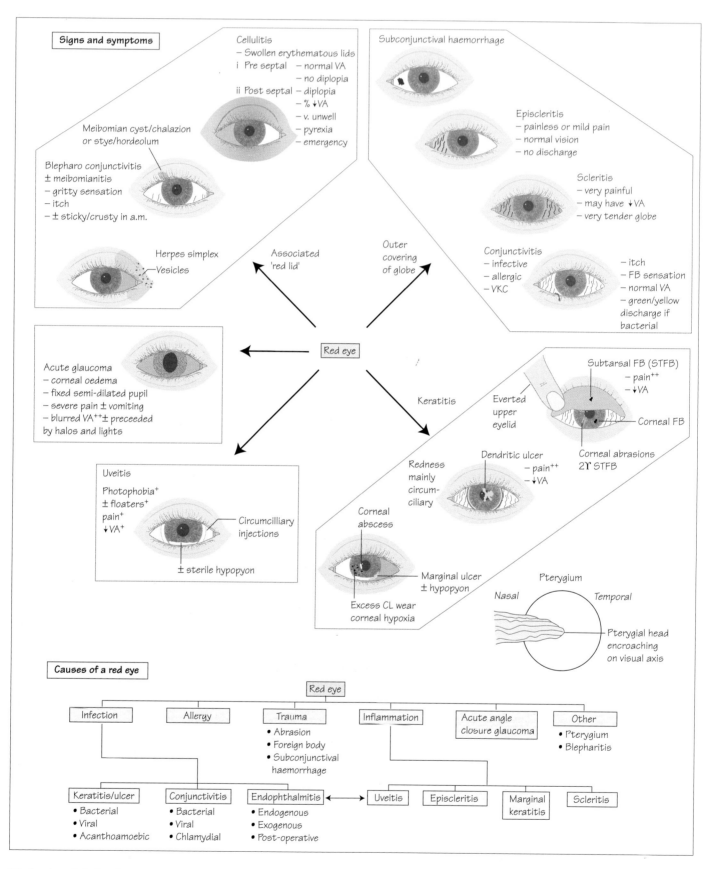

Signs and symptoms

Cellulitis
– Swollen erythematous lids
i Pre septal – normal VA
 – no diplopia
ii Post septal – diplopia
 – % ↓VA
 – v. unwell
 – pyrexia
 – emergency

Subconjunctival haemorrhage

Episcleritis
– painless or mild pain
– normal vision
– no discharge

Meibomian cyst/chalazion or stye/hordeolum

Blepharo conjunctivitis
± meibomianitis
– gritty sensation
– itch
– ± sticky/crusty in a.m.

Scleritis
– very painful
– may have ↓VA
– very tender globe

Herpes simplex
– Vesicles

Conjunctivitis
– infective
– allergic
– VKC

– itch
– FB sensation
– normal VA
– green/yellow discharge if bacterial

Associated 'red lid'

Outer covering of globe

Acute glaucoma
– corneal oedema
– fixed semi-dilated pupil
– severe pain ± vomiting
– blurred VA⁺⁺± preceded by halos and lights

Red eye

Keratitis

Subtarsal FB (STFB)
– pain⁺⁺
– ↓VA

Everted upper eyelid

Corneal FB

Corneal abrasions
2⁰ STFB

Uveitis
Photophobia⁺
± floaters⁺
pain⁺
↓VA⁺

Circumcilliary injections

± sterile hypopyon

Redness mainly circumciliary

Dendritic ulcer
– pain⁺⁺
– ↓VA

Corneal abscess

Marginal ulcer ± hypopyon

Excess CL wear corneal hypoxia

Pterygium

Nasal   Temporal

Pterygial head encroaching on visual axis

Causes of a red eye

Red eye

| Infection | Allergy | Trauma | Inflammation | Acute angle closure glaucoma | Other |

Trauma:
• Abrasion
• Foreign body
• Subconjunctival haemorrhage

Other:
• Pterygium
• Blepharitis

| Keratitis/ulcer | Conjunctivitis | Endophthalmitis | ↔ | Uveitis | Episcleritis | Marginal keratitis | Scleritis |

Keratitis/ulcer:
• Bacterial
• Viral
• Acanthoamoebic

Conjunctivitis:
• Bacterial
• Viral
• Chlamydial

Endophthalmitis:
• Endogenous
• Exogenous
• Post-operative

Allergic conjunctivitis (see Chapter 29)

Symptoms
- Itchy red eye in patient who may have a history of atopy (e.g. asthma, eczema, hay fever).

Signs
- Diffuse or localized conjunctival injection.
- Chemosis, normal vision.

Treatment
- Topical mast cell stabilizer and antihistamine bd (such as Opatanol or Zaditen).
- Topical steroids initially if severe.
- Vernal keratoconjunctivitis sicca (VKC): treat as for allergic and refer to an ophthalmic unit.

Subconjunctival haemorrhage (SCH)

Symptoms
- Sudden onset of painless red eye.
- Occasionally patient says he 'felt something give' or 'pop'.

Signs
- Localized dense red haemmorhage on an otherwise normal eye.

Treatment
- Reassure it will resolve spontaneously.
- Ask patient about excessive straining such as severe coughing or vomiting which can cause SCH—usually bilateral.
- Check blood pressure, full blood count (FBC) and blood glucose.

Episcleritis

Symptoms
- Red eye.
- Usually painless, or can have mild dull pain.

Signs
- Localized or diffuse episcleral injection.
- Non-tender.
- Normal vision.
- No discharge.

Treatment
- G Voltarol qds.
- Rarely systemic indomethacin.

Scleritis

Symptoms
- Extremely painful red eye.
- May have blurred vision.

Signs
- Intense injection of the scleral and episcleral vessels.
- Globe extremely tender.

Treatment
- Rule out systemic disease, e.g. rheumatoid arthritis.

- *Non-necrotizing*: Treat with systemic indomethacin 100 mg od for 4 days, then reduce to 75 mg po od until inflammation is resolved.
- *Necrotizing*: high dose immunosupression.

Blepharitis/meibomianitis

Signs and symptoms
See Chapter 29.

Treatment
- Lid hygiene bd.
- G fucithalmic bd for up to 3 months.
- Topical lubricant six times per day.
- Review after 3 months, if no improvement add minocycline 100 mg bd for 3 months.

Meibomian cyst or chalazion/stye or hordeolum (see Chapters 23 and 24)

Treatment
- G chloromycetin hourly for 3 days, qds for 10 days.
- Hot compresses and remove lash if there is a stye.
- If early pre-septal cellulitis, add systemic antibiotics for 10 days.

Orbital cellulitis
Signs, symptoms and management. See Chapter 23.

Primary herpes simplex infection of eyelids

Symptoms
Sore red eye and eyelid usually in a child.

Signs
Vesicles on lids in early stages—eschar in later stages.

Treatment
- Occ aciclovir five times per day for 1 week, then tds for 1 week, bd for 1 week, od for 1 week and then stop.
- Exclude corneal involvement with fluorescein.

Pterygium (see Chapter 32)

Symptoms
Localized redness medially, irritation +/– blurred vision.

Signs
Wing-shaped abnormal growths of conjunctival-derived fibrovascular tissue. Inflammation and blurred vision due to visual axis obstruction or astigmatism.

Aetiology
Subconjunctival elastotic degeneration from UV damage and dryness, e.g. Australia and other dry desert equatorial countries.

Treatment
- Medical—topical lubricants +/– G Volterol.
- Surgical—excision and conjunctival autografts.
    - β-irradiation or antimetabolites applied perioperatively in recurrence.

15 Ophthalmic trauma principles and management of chemical injuries

Medicolegal considerations

Meticulous history recording, clinical examination, visual acuity recording, note taking and photographs of the injuries are required. All trauma cases should be regarded as potential medicolegal cases especially when an alleged assault has taken place or it has been an occupational injury. Always sign your name clearly and date and time the clinical notes accurately

The principles of trauma apply:
- Airway
- Breathing
- Cardiovascular

Once these are stabilized the ophthalmologist is asked to examine the orbital / eye injury

Ophthalmic trauma is:
- Chemical–Emergency
- Blunt
- Sharp and perforating

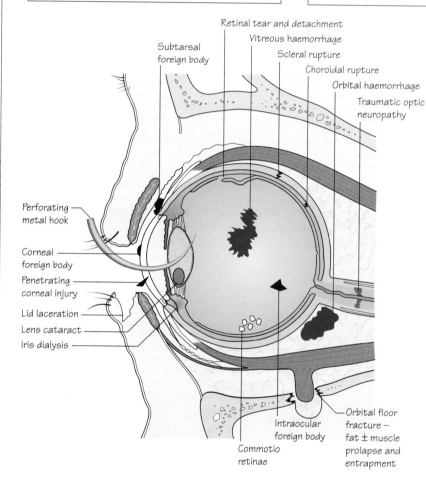

Retinal tear and detachment
Vitreous haemorrhage
Scleral rupture
Choroidal rupture
Orbital haemorrhage
Traumatic optic neuropathy

Subtarsal foreign body

Perforating metal hook
Corneal foreign body
Penetrating corneal injury
Lid laceration
Lens cataract
Iris dialysis

Intraocular foreign body
Commotio retinae
Orbital floor fracture – fat ± muscle prolapse and entrapment

How to wash out a chemical injury

This is the only occasion when you wash out the eye first then measure the visual acuity second. It is an emergency!

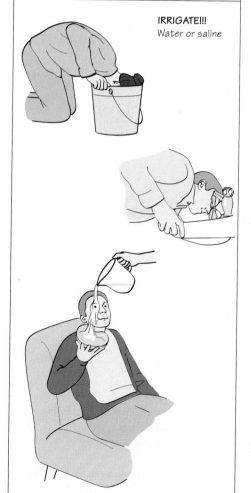

IRRIGATE!!!
Water or saline

Examination

- Take a thorough history and record exactly what happened
- Measure the visual acuity (in chemical injury can do after washout)
- Examine the eye systematically from the outside lids to the retina, incuding pupil reactions
- **Dilate pupils for fundal examination**
- ± Radiological investigation
- Photograph for medicolegal purposes

Aims

1 List the main causes of loss of vision due to trauma.
2 How to wash out a chemical injury.

Principles of ophthalmic trauma

Basic ophthalmic trauma knowledge is required in the accident and emergency setting, in intensive care and in the primary eye care clinic. The trauma patient may be managed by plastics and maxillofacial surgeons if there are facial or orbital fractures, or neurosurgeons if there is a head injury.

The five main causes of loss of vision with trauma are:

1 Corneal scarring and anterior segment damage from severe alkali burn.
2 Severe disrupted globe from penetrating injury, e.g. road traffic accident.
3 Unrecognized intraocular metallic foreign body causing siderosis bulbi.
4 Compressive optic neuropathy from retrobulbar haemorrhage.
5 Traumatic optic neuropathy from optic canal bony or shearing injury.

Trauma can affect the periocular region, bony orbit, orbital contents, globe or optic nerve.

1 Eyelid and periocular and orbital haematoma—fully assess to rule out orbital floor fracture and fracture of base of skull
2 Orbital bony wall fracture—floor > medial wall with diplopia, needs repair
3 Eyelid subtarsal foreign body—evert lid and remove with cotton bud
4 Eyelids—partial or full thickness laceration: explore wound, exclude penetrating eye injury and repair within 48 h
5 Lacrimal drainage system—most commonly lower canaliculus; needs oculoplastics repair and stent, e.g. MiniMonaka tube
6 Conjunctival laceration—may need suturing; exclude more extensive deeper injury
7 Corneal abrasion—treat with topical antibiotics ± cycloplegia and a pad
8 Corneal foreign body—needs removal and dilated fundoscopy
9 Corneal penetrating injury ± sclera, iris, lens or retinal injury—all require urgent surgical repair
10 Hypahaema (blood in the anterior chamber)—can cause secondary glaucoma; needs urgent ophthalmic assessment
11 Dislocated lens—may need surgery to remove lens
12 Traumatic cataract—most need surgical removal
13 Glaucoma secondary to angle recession (i.e. damage to trabecular meshwork)—needs specialist treatment
14 Blunt vitreous haemorrhage and retinal commotio—needs vitreoretinal assessment to exclude retinal tear
15 Retinal tear/dialysis—needs urgent retinal surgery
16 Choroidal rupture—may lose vision if underlies macula; untreatable
17 Scleral perforation—needs surgical exploration and repair; if extensive may loose eye (enucleation)
18 Massive retrobulbar haemorrhage—needs urgent lateral canthotomy/cantholysis to decompress orbit
19 Traumatic optic neuropathy—needs to be treated with high dose steroids within hours
20 Traumatic cranial nerve injury—IVth, IIIrd and VIth cranial nerves need MRI scan
21 Complete globe disruption—needs enucleation within 14 days to prevent sympathetic ophthalmia

If any of the above are suspected refer *immediately* to eye casualty

---

Chemical injuries

Which chemical? Substances include alkalis (lime, cement, plaster or ammonia), acids, solvents, detergents, irritants (e.g. mace and pepper) and super-glue. Alkalis (e.g. ammonia or wet cement) are the most destructive, penetrating the deep layers of the eye with time. In high concentrations they cause severe ischaemia of the conjunctiva, corneal limbus, cornea and sclera, and cause subsequent scarring and blindness. There may be associated severe uveitis and cataract formation. *Wash out the eye immediately!*

1 Measure the pH of the tear meniscus if litmus paper is handy.
2 Otherwise, apply immediately topical anaesthetic drops if handy.
3 Copious irrigation with normal saline or Ringer's solution. If neither are available, put the patient's head under a cold water tap or into a bowl of cold water—with eyes open! Irrigate/splash the eyes for 5–10 min, then repeat the pH measurement.
4 Ensure that the surface of the eye and the upper and lower fornices are included. Using a cotton bud, evert the upper lid and check for fragments of cement, etc. and remove them. Swipe the cotton bud along the lower fornix to remove particulate debris.
5 Now measure the visual acuity and check the eye, including intra-ocular pressure.
6 Admit.
7 Topical treatment: intensive topical antibiotics, vitamin C and cycloplegia (to prevent pain) ± steroids. Treat raised intra-ocular pressure as necessary.
8 Oral high dose vitamin C.
9 Later surgery if need—limbal cell transplant and penetrating keratoplasty (corneal graft).

KEY POINTS

- All trauma cases are medicolegal cases until proved otherwise.
- Ocular trauma is chemical, blunt or sharp (perforating).
- Alkali burns can cause blindness and must be irrigated immediately.

16 Specific features of blunt and sharp injuries

Blunt injuries

Small hyphaema

Blackball

3 mm

Sphincter pupil ruptures

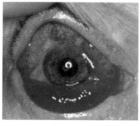
Subconjunctival haemorrhage and chemosis

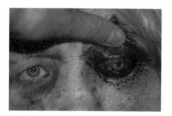
Acute massive orbital haemorrhage with proptosis

NB May need urgent lateral cantholysis and canthotomy to drain a traumatic retrobulbar haemorrhage

Retinal and choroidal blunt injury

Choroidal rupture (yellow-white streak)

Commotio retinae (white)

Commotio retinae is likely to recover but the rarer choroidal rupture can persist and, if on the macula, cause severe decreased vision

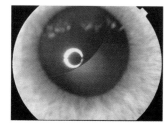
Dislocated lens

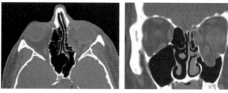
CT scan of left orbital medial wall and floor fracture – patient has severe enophthalmos and diplopia from restricted eye movement

WARNING

Exclude small entry wound of an intraocular foreign body (IOFB). Dilate the pupil and examine the fundus to exclude IOFB. If there is a history of hammering, use orbital X-ray to exclude IOFB

Sharp injuries

Corneal foreign bodies

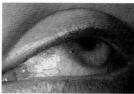

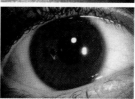

Remove with a cotton bud or sharp needle with good illumination and magnification. May leave a rust ring which needs later further removal with a needle

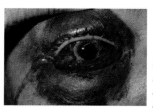
Severe ocular trauma with a corneo-scleral rupture, lens disclocation, retinal detachment and vitreous haemorrhage

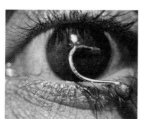
Corneal perforation with fishing hook – may have perforated lens

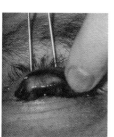
Double eversion of upper eyelid

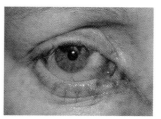
Medial eyelid and lacrimal canaliculus avulsion. Needs primary repair and canalicular intubation

Subtarsal foreign body

Scratch marks on cornea lightly staining

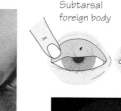

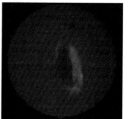
Intraocular foreign body Needs vitrectomy and removal

Anterior segment sharp injury

Lens perforation

Axial corneal full thickness laceration

Iris pulled up to wound

Corneoscleral laceration

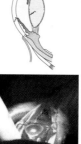
Exploratory microsurgery is indicated to determine the extent of the globe rupture and to carry out a primary repair

Aims

1 How to manage a retrobulbar haemorrhage.
2 How to remove a corneal foreign body.
3 How to manage a corneal abrasion.

Blunt injuries

From a fist/cricket/squash/tennis ball/champagne cork, etc.
• Causes lid echymosis, orbital and subconjunctival haematoma, hyphaema, ± lens iris injury, vitreous haemorrhage and commotio retinae.
• Look for associated conjunctival and corneal foreign bodies, abrasions and lacerations and a red reflex.
• Exclude traumatic emphysema from bony fracture—rare.
• Exclude a perforating ocular injury, traumatic retinal detachment or optic neuropathy (vision will be markedly reduced with an afferent pupil defect and normal optic disc).
• Exclude orbital floor fracture by examining eye movements and for infraorbital numbness. If a fracture is suspected arrange an orbital CT scan.

The following are the main blunt injuries seen.

Traumatic hyphaema

This is blood in the anterior chamber. It can be microscopic (seen only on slit lamp), or it can form a level, the height of which is measured in millimetres, or it can be a complete blackball. Causes pain and blurred vision.

Traumatic iritis

White cells and flare in the anterior chamber (seen only on slit lamp), causing dull pain and photophobia.

Orbital haematoma

• **Eyelid echymosis.** There are usually superficial lacerations causing the bleeding. Insert a topical anaesthetic drop to help open the eye gently and measure the visual acuity, examine the eye movements, exclude a perforating eye injury and look at the fundus.
• **Retrobulbar haemorrhage.** This is potentially sight-threatening. There is pain, decreased vision, proptosis and diffuse subconjunctival haemorrhage extending posteriorly. It can follow periocular infiltrative anaesthesia or blunt trauma (with orbital wall fracture) and be associated with a ruptured globe and carotid-cavernous sinus fistula. Emergency lateral canthotomy and cantholysis is necessary to relieve high orbital pressure and to reduce the risk of compressive optic neuropathy.

Retinal bruising (commotio retinae)

Blurred vision can occur due to retinal bruising and loss of central vision from a choroidal rupture across the macula.

Traumatic optic neuropathy

This may respond to high dose steroids or optic canal decompression.

Orbital floor fracture

Blow-out fracture of the floor or medial wall into the sinus. Orbital soft tissue entrapment may cause diplopia and limited eye movements. Enophthalmos may not be immediately apparent until swelling/haemorrhage has settled.

Sharp, penetrating and perforating injuries

Sharp objects, e.g. glass, spiky plant, hammer and chisal, cause eyelid, corneoscleral, iris, lens and retinal lacerations. Often, though, the entry wound is small and a high index of suspicion should therefore exist for hammering and other high velocity injuries. Perforating injuries require urgent exploration and repair by the on-duty ophthalmologist. The vitreo-retinal and oculoplastics surgeons work closely together with these patients. Sometimes the eye must be enucleated when the injury is very severe.

> **TIPS**
> • Do not put pressure on an eye that may be perforated or contents may extrude!
> • X-ray for suspected intraocular foreign body.

Superficial corneal injuries

Corneal foreign bodies (FBs) and subtarsal foreign bodies (STFBs). History of a particle entering the eye, either dust or metal flying in whilst walking past a building site, grinding metal/hammering/doing DIY.

Symptoms
• Painful photophobic red watering eye—worse for corneal FBs than STFBs.

Signs
• Corneal FB sits embedded superficially on corneal epithelium.
• STFB lies embedded on the upper tarsal conjunctiva and causes typical superior corneal superficial epithelial abrasions.

Management
• Use topical anaesthesia to examine. Instil fluorescein drops to help see the FB and epithelial scratches from the STFB.
• Try and flick the corneal FB off with a cotton bud. If it is too embedded, the ophthalmologist can use a sharp needle end to remove it at the slit lamp.
• Evert the upper eyelid to see and remove the STFB with a cotton bud wiped across it. Immediate symptomatic relief.
• Instil topical antibiotics, cycloplegic drops and pad for 24 h, then a short course of topical antibiotics.

Corneal abrasion

History of scratch from a sharp plant, paper, child's finger nail, etc.

Symptoms
Severe pain and FB sensation, photophobia and watering.

Signs
Red eye with fluorescein staining epithelial abrasion.

Management
• Use topical anaesthesia to examine.
• Instil fluorescein to show abrasion clearly with blue light.
• Pad with a cycloplegic drop and topical antibiotic.

Sharp objects heal initially but later can cause symptoms of nocturnal and early morning FB sensation—called recurrent erosion syndrome (RES).

KEY POINTS
• Retrobulbar haemorrhage— canthotomy + cantholysis saves vision.
• Evert the upper eyelid to remove a subtarsal foreign body with a cotton bud.
• Corneal abrasion from a sharp object can cause RES.

17 Sudden painful loss of vision in a non-inflamed eye

Sudden painful loss of vision

Sudden loss of vision associated with eye pain or headache in the white non-inflamed eye needs urgent attention as it may be due to sight or even life-threatening illness. The frequency of each disease varies between age groups

Giant cell arteritis (GCA)

GCA – inflammation of the lining of large and medium sized arteries. Immediate treatment with corticosteroids usually relieves symptoms and prevents loss of vision

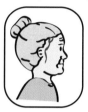

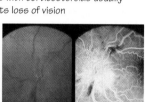

Swollen disc of arteritic anterior ischaemic optic neuropathy – colour and fluorescein angiogram appearance

- Elderly patient
- Non pulsatile tender temporal artery
- ± Headache (may be painless)
- ± Jaw claudication
- ± Weight loss
- High ESR and CRP

Haemorrhage from pituitary tumour

Pituitary tumour

- May involve one optic nerve or tract causing sudden vision loss

Migraine

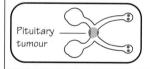

- Fortification spectra

- May see zigzag lines
- Can lose vision temporarily

Scintillating scotoma

Cast of blood supply of human eye Copyright J Olver

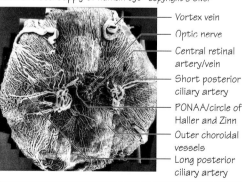

- Vortex vein
- Optic nerve
- Central retinal artery/vein
- Short posterior ciliary artery
- PONAA/circle of Haller and Zinn
- Outer choroidal vessels
- Long posterior ciliary artery

1 mm
30 mm
1 mm

Left altitudinal field defect typical of anterior ischaemic optic neuropathy

Optic neuritis/retrobulbar neuritis

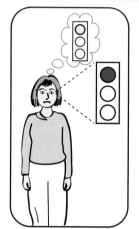

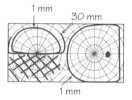

May have swollen optic nerve or look normal if retrobulbar neuritis (i.e. inflammation behind globe)

- Young woman
- Pain on eye movement

Benign intracranial hypertension (BIH)

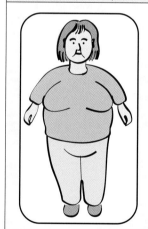

- Usually overweight females (though can occur in slim adults and children of either sex)
- Causes progressive field loss but also sudden visual loss in the form of transient visual obscurations (TVOs)

- Fields showing constriction. Shaded area is where target is not visualized

Aetiology of optic neuritis

- Typical: Idiopathic
  Multiple sclerosis is the most common cause of retrobulbar neuritis
- Atypical: Infectious (viral)
  Post infectious
  Granulomatous
  Autoimmune
  Contiguous inflammation of orbit, sinuses or meninges

Aim

1 Identify the main causes of sudden painful loss of vision in a white eye.
2 Note that the pain may be ocular or cranial or both.

Giant cell arteritis (GCA)/Temporal arteritis

This is visual disturbance with headache in elderly patients. This inflammatory condition can result in occlusion of the larger blood vessels supplying the anterior optic nerve leading to anterior ischaemic optic neuropathy (AION); this is referred to as **arteritic AION** when the aetiology is GCA. There is also a **non-arteritic AION** which is painless and is caused by occlusion or hypoperfusion within the smaller blood vessels supplying the optic nerve, the circle of Haller and Zinn (see figure of cast, opposite).

- In arteritic AION the patient is usually elderly and complains of:
  —sudden loss of vision, which may only affect the upper or lower half of the visual field (altitudinal visual field defect);
  —headache (not always present).
  —sometimes a recent history of pain in the cheeks when chewing—jaw claudication;
  —often a recent history of weight loss, myalgia and arthralgia.
- On examination there may be temporal artery tenderness.
- If there is associated chest pain suspect coronary artery involvement, which may lead to cardiac infarction and death if not treated.
- Inflammation of the cerebral vessels can lead to a cerebrovascular accident (CVA).
- Patients with GCA often have a high ESR, and invariably an elevated CRP (though both may be normal initially).
- Definitive diagnosis is by temporal artery biopsy. This is best done within a few days of commencing steroids.
- Treatment, which must be swift in order to prevent blindness, is with high dose steroids and requires hospital admission. Treatment must not be delayed whilst waiting for a biopsy; once a clinical diagnosis is made, instigate treatment immediately.
- Patients with this condition may be on steroids for several years and must be put on calcium and a biphosphonate (to reduce osteoporosis), and a proton pump inhibitor. They must have their weight, blood pressure and blood glucose monitored.

Optic neuritis/retrobulbar neuritis

This is visual disturbance with eye pain.
- Inflammation of the optic nerve. If the entire anterior part of the nerve is inflamed, the optic disc will appear swollen (papillitis).
- **Retrobulbar neuritis** (RBN): If the part of the nerve behind the globe (i.e. the retrobulbar part of the nerve) is affected, with sparing of the nerve head, the patient will have the same symptoms with reduced visual acuity, red desaturation and a relative afferent papillary defect, but the disc will appear normal in the acute phase.

  Typical optic neuritis/retrobulbar neuritis:
- Most commonly affects young adults.
- Females affected more than males.
- Patient presents with:
  —sudden loss of vision—this may vary from complete loss of vision to alteration in colour perception (e.g. the patient may complain of colours looking 'washed out' with the affected eye);

  —there is often associated eye pain, particularly induced by eye movement.
- Typically, the vision improves over a period of 4–6 weeks, though this is not always the case.
- There may be other symptoms attributable to demyelination, such as paraesthesia, bladder or bowel dysfuntion, and limb weakness.
- There may have been a recent viral illness.
- The diagnosis of optic or retrobulbar neuritis can be aided by performing visual evoked potential (VEP), which will demonstrate increased latency, i.e. a 'delayed response'.
- MRI also helps to confirm the diagnosis, as the affected nerve lights up, and it will show up demyelinating plaques in the brain.
- In most centres systemic steroid therapy for optic neuritis is reserved for bilateral cases; as although it has been shown to speed up visual recovery, it has not been demonstrated to improve final visual outcome.

Migraine

This is visual disturbance with headache.
These visual disturbances most commonly present as fortification spectra or scintillating scotoma, but occasionally as field loss or even total loss of vision, which recovers. There is often a family history of migraine.

Idiopathic intracranial hypertension (IIH) or benign intracranial hypertension (BIH)

Presents with headache and transient visual obscurations (TVOs). TVOs last for a few seconds, are unilateral or bilateral, and are usually precipitated by movement or postural changes. They are pathognomonic of papilloedema.
- Occurs typically in obese females, but can affect slim individuals of either sex, and children.
- The optic discs are swollen and there is field loss.
- An MRI should be performed to exclude a space-occupying lesion and an MRA to exclude venous sinus thrombosis, or an arteriovenous malformation affecting the venous sinuses.
- Thyroid dysfunction is a cause and must be excluded.
- Patients should be referred for urgent treatment, as this disease often results in permanent loss of the visual field.
- Treatment includes:
  —conservative: weight loss; stop any medications that may cause BIH (e.g. NSAIDs, tetracyclines);
  —medical: acetazolamide;
  —surgical: lumbo- or ventriculo-peritoneal shunt, or optic nerve sheath fenestration.

Haemorrhage associated with pituitary tumour

Rarely, a small haemorrhage into an undiagnosed pituitary tumour can cause sudden loss of vision associated with headache. Such patients require *urgent* referral to a neurosurgical unit, as this is a precursor of pituitary apoplexy.

KEY POINTS
- Painful loss of vision in a quiet eye may have a systemic cause, e.g. giant cell arteritis.
- Retrobulbar neuritis — the disc looks normal in the acute phase.
- Idiopathic intracranial hypertension — the discs are swollen.

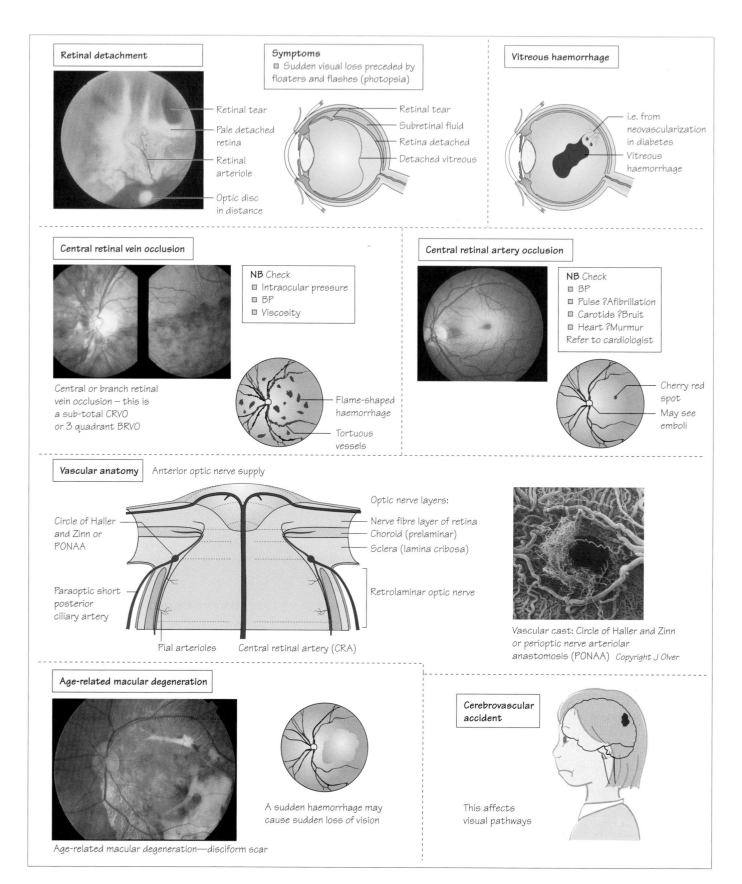

Retinal detachment
- Retinal tear
- Pale detached retina
- Retinal arteriole
- Optic disc in distance

Symptoms
- Sudden visual loss preceded by floaters and flashes (photopsia)
- Retinal tear
- Subretinal fluid
- Retina detached
- Detached vitreous

Vitreous haemorrhage
- i.e. from neovascularization in diabetes
- Vitreous haemorrhage

Central retinal vein occlusion

Central or branch retinal vein occlusion – this is a sub-total CRVO or 3 quadrant BRVO

NB Check
- Intraocular pressure
- BP
- Viscosity

- Flame-shaped haemorrhage
- Tortuous vessels

Central retinal artery occlusion

NB Check
- BP
- Pulse ?Afibrillation
- Carotids ?Bruit
- Heart ?Murmur
Refer to cardiologist

- Cherry red spot
- May see emboli

Vascular anatomy | Anterior optic nerve supply

- Circle of Haller and Zinn or PONAA
- Paraoptic short posterior ciliary artery
- Pial arterioles
- Central retinal artery (CRA)

Optic nerve layers:
- Nerve fibre layer of retina
- Choroid (prelaminar)
- Sclera (lamina cribosa)
- Retrolaminar optic nerve

Vascular cast: Circle of Haller and Zinn or perioptic nerve arteriolar anastomosis (PONAA) Copyright J Olver

Age-related macular degeneration

Age-related macular degeneration—disciform scar

A sudden haemorrhage may cause sudden loss of vision

Cerebrovascular accident

This affects visual pathways

Aim

Identify the main causes of painless loss of vision, in particular:
- retinal detachment;
- vitreous haemorrhage;
- types of vascular occlusion.

Retinal detachment (see Chapter 39)

- Sudden (sometimes gradual) painless loss of vision.
- Usually preceded by symptoms of flashing lights (photopsia) and/or floaters and/or visual field defects.
- When the macula is not involved the visual loss involves the peripheral field and visual acuity may be normal.
- Once the macula is involved the central vision is lost.

Management
Laser to retinal hole or retinal surgery ± vitrectomy.

Vitreous haemorrhage

Haemorrhage into the vitreous cavity can result in sudden painless loss of vision. The extent of visual loss will depend on the degree of haemorrhage.
- A large haemorrhage will cause total visual loss
- A small haemorrhage will present as floaters and normal or only slightly reduced visual acuity.
  Aetiology:
- Proliferative retinopathy—spontaneous rupture of abnormal fragile new vessels that grow on the retinal surface cause bleeding into the vitreous cavity. Most common is proliferative diabetic retinopathy.
- Retinal detachment—a small retinal blood vessel may rupture when the retinal break occurs, bleeding into the vitreous cavity.
- Trauma.
- Posterior vitreous detachment (see Chapter 39 for details) can result in vitreous haemorrhage if, as the vitreous separates from the retina, it pulls and ruptures a small blood vessel.
- Age-related macula degeneration (AMD)—haemorrhage may occur into the vitreous from the abnormally weak vessels forming a subretinal neovascular membrane (see Chapter 41).

Management
Referral to an ophthalmologist to determine cause and manage any complications (e.g. glaucoma due to red blood cells clogging up trabecular meshwork) that may occur.

Vascular occlusion (see Chapters 44 and 45)

Central retinal vein occlusion (CRVO) or a branch retinal vein occlusion (BRVO) often presents with sudden painless loss of vision. Aetiology:
- Systemic hypertension.
- Raised intraocular pressure.
- Hyperviscosity syndromes.
- Vessel wall disease (e.g. diabetes, inflammation such as sarcoidosis).

> **WARNING**
> - All patients with vein occlusion must have their blood pressure checked, should be examined for arteriosclerosis, have their intraocular pressure checked and be checked for diabetes and systemic inflammation.
> - Young patients presenting with CRVO or BRVO, or older patients in whom there is no obvious cause, should be fully checked out for hyperviscosity syndromes.

Central retinal artery occlusion (CRAO) or a branch retinal artery occlusion also presents as acute painless loss of vision. Aetiology:
- Very high intraocular pressure, as seen in acute angle closure glaucoma.
- Arterial embolus from diseased carotid, valvular heart disease, atrial fibrillation.
- Arterial occlusion from atheroma or inflammation (e.g. giant cell arteritis).

> **WARNING**
> All patients with CRAO need full cardiovascular work-up.

Non-arteritic anterior (AION) or posterior ischaemic optic neuropathy (PION):
- Results from occlusion or hypoperfusion of the small blood vessels supplying the optic nerve head (AION) or posterior optic nerve (PION).
- In AION the optic disc is swollen; this swelling may be segmental or involve the entire nerve head. There are usually associated splinter haemorrhages at the disc.
- In PION the optic disc looks normal.
- There may be arteriosclerosis and arteriovenous nipping, depending on the cause.
- Risk factors: arteriosclerosis, hypertension, hypotensive episode, smoking, 'disc at risk' (e.g. small optic nerve head with no central cup).

Cerebrovascular accident (CVA)

A haemorrhagic or embolic CVA affecting the visual pathways will present as acute painless visual loss. Depending on the site of the lesion, the patient will have a corresponding field defect on fields to confrontation. (See Chapter 50.)

Acephalgic migraine

This rare form of migraine presents with transient visual disturbances involving one or both eyes in the absence of headaches.

KEY POINTS
1 Retinal detachment is an ocular cause of sudden painless loss of vision.
2 Central retinal vein occlusion is commonly caused by systemic hypertension.
3 Central retinal artery occlusion may be caused by giant cell arteritis.

19 Gradual loss of vision

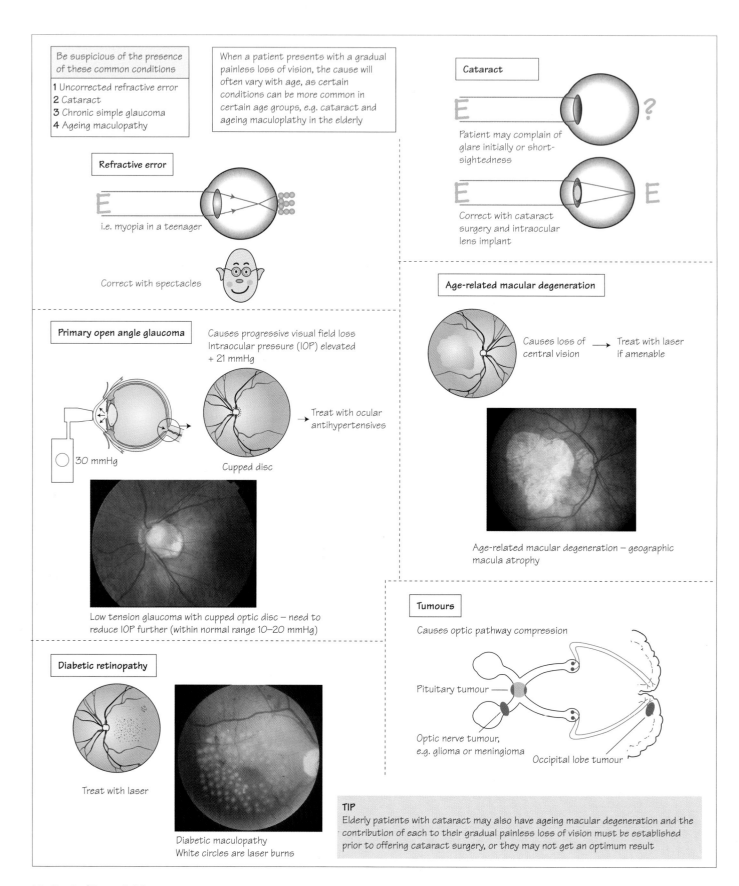

Be suspicious of the presence of these common conditions

1 Uncorrected refractive error
2 Cataract
3 Chronic simple glaucoma
4 Ageing maculopathy

When a patient presents with a gradual painless loss of vision, the cause will often vary with age, as certain conditions can be more common in certain age groups, e.g. cataract and ageing maculoplathy in the elderly

Refractive error

i.e. myopia in a teenager

Correct with spectacles

Cataract

Patient may complain of glare initially or short-sightedness

Correct with cataract surgery and intraocular lens implant

Primary open angle glaucoma

Causes progressive visual field loss
Intraocular pressure (IOP) elevated + 21 mmHg

30 mmHg

Cupped disc

Treat with ocular antihypertensives

Low tension glaucoma with cupped optic disc – need to reduce IOP further (within normal range 10–20 mmHg)

Age-related macular degeneration

Causes loss of central vision → Treat with laser if amenable

Age-related macular degeneration – geographic macula atrophy

Diabetic retinopathy

Treat with laser

Diabetic maculopathy
White circles are laser burns

Tumours

Causes optic pathway compression

Pituitary tumour

Optic nerve tumour, e.g. glioma or meningioma

Occipital lobe tumour

TIP
Elderly patients with cataract may also have ageing macular degeneration and the contribution of each to their gradual painless loss of vision must be established prior to offering cataract surgery, or they may not get an optimum result

Aim

Easily identify the common causes of gradual painless loss of vision in a white eye.

Refractive error

Undetected and uncorrected refractive error is a common cause of gradual visual loss in all age groups. Hypermetropia occurs in young children, axial myopia in teenagers and young adults, and lenticular myopia in older patients.

• Early cataract formation (nuclear sclerosis) may induce a refractive error (most commonly myopia) in the elderly—they are briefly happy because they discard their glasses for reading! However, their distance visual acuity gradually deteriorates and they require surgery.

• Children with refractive errors don't complain until they attend school and have difficulty seeing the blackboard (myopia) or the print in their text books (hypermetropia or astigmatism), or complain of headaches at the end of the day due to eye strain (asthenopia). The child often doesn't complain at all, and it is the teacher who notices a problem. Unfortunately, for some children with hypermetropia, amblyopia has already occurred in one eye by the time the diagnosis is made and despite full refractive error correction with glasses and patching, vision in one eye does not improve. (See Chapters 9 and 21).

Cataract

• A common cause of gradual loss of vision in the elderly. They may notice nothing at all and the presence of an early cataract is detected by their optician or they will have a gradual blurring of distant, then near, vision. If the cataract is placed posterior in the lens as a plaque (posterior sub-capsular lens opacity) they will notice glare and reduced vision in bright sunlight with improved vision indoors.

• It may also occur in younger age groups who are at risk (e.g. patient with diabetes, patients on steroids, patients with chronic uveitis and those with a family history of cataract).

• Cataract may also occur in young children (congenital cataract). It is very important to check the red reflex of any child who presents with reduced vision, and any baby who does not fix and follow, as they require urgent treatment with patching and glasses to prevent amblyopia. (See Chapter 21).

Primary open-angle glaucoma (POAG) (chronic simple)

Causes slowly progressive painless visual field loss.
• It is most commonly seen in adults over 40 years of age, though it can occur in younger adults.
• Risk factors include Afro-Caribbean origin, family history of primary open angle glaucoma and hypertension.
• The patient is usually completely unaware that they have open angle glaucoma and it is detected by their optician finding raised intraocular pressure or noticing a cupped disc.
• By the time a patient with glaucoma presents with visual symptoms, the optic disc will show evidence of damage and be very cupped (end-stage disease).

Glaucoma screening will often pick up POAG before any severe damage has occurred and many patients are maintained on topical medication without significant progression or the need for drainage surgery (see Chapters 36–38).

Retinal disease

Should be considered in the patient with none of the above causes of reduced vision. It occurs particularly in patients at risk:
• Patients with diabetes (diabetic retinopathy).
• Patients with hypertension (hypertensive retinopathy).
• The elderly (age-related macular degeneration, ARMD). This is the commonest cause of blindness in the elderly, in which their central vision for reading, colour and fine detail is affected. They cannot see people's faces or expressions clearly or read the labels on food in the supermarket or read the newspaper.
• Children or young adults with neurometabolic diseases or a family history of retinal disease (e.g. retinitis pigmentosa).
• An individual with a history of an intraocular foreign body (IOFB) may develop siderosis bulbi; this is a condition where iron from an IOFB that has not been removed can cause retinal toxicity. The patient presents years after the initial injury with gradual loss of vision. The iris in the affected eye of a blue-eyed individual may have a greenish hue.
• Individuals taking medications known to cause drug-induced macular disease (e.g. chloroquine, hydroxychloroquine, tamoxifen, chlorpromazine, thioridazine, vigabatrin).

Tumours and inflammation

Any tumour that affects the visual pathway may cause symptoms of gradual, painless loss of vision by pressure on the optic nerve or eye. Examples include:
• Intraocular tumour (e.g. choroidal malignant melanoma or choroidal metastases from the breast or prostate in adults, retinoblastoma in children)
• Intraocular lymphoma, which may masquerade as bilateral uveitis.
• Tumour of the optic nerve (e.g. meningioma or glioma).
• Tumour of the orbit or optic nerve (e.g. orbital lymphoma, sphenoidal wing meningioma, dysthyroid eye disease).
• Any brain tumour involving the visual pathways (e.g. pituitary tumour, occipital lobe tumour).
These are not common and should always be considered when no other cause can be found.

KEY POINTS
• Myopia is common in young teenagers.
• Patients with POAG are usually unaware of their disease.
• Cataract and ageing maculopathy cause decreased vision in the elderly.
• Tumours are a rare cause.

Newborn up to 2 months old

1. Fix and follow. In the newborn see if they will fix and follow a shiny colourful target

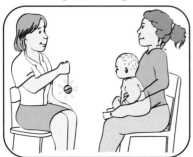

2. Spinning. Another way of getting a crude idea of vision is to pick the child up, and hold him at arm's length and spin him around in a circle

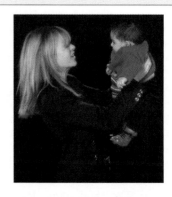

3. More advanced ways of checking a newborn's vision include forced choice preferential looking (FPL or PL), a clinical test

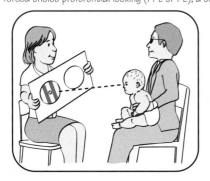

4. Electrophysiological testing with visual evoked potentials (VEPs) /visual evoked responses (VERs)

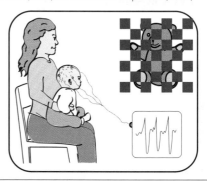

Infant and toddler up to 3 years old

In the pre-verbal infant, vision can be assessed as for the newborn. Older infants can see pictures of familiar objects (fish, apple, boat)

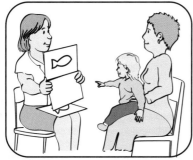

Cardiff Acuity Cards
– best for infants

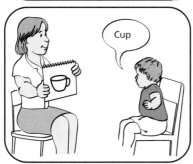

Kay Pictures
– best for toddlers

4 to 5 year olds

Depending on social background and learning ability most 4 and 5 year olds will be able to match letters, and some children at this age can even read letters. For children who cannot read letters the "Sheridan–Gardner singles" test is used

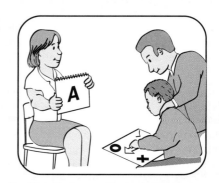

Sheridan–Gardner singles

Aim

How to assess visual acuity in different aged children.

Visual development

A child's vision continues to develop after birth and maturation does not fully occur until after age 2 years. Normal visual development in both eyes is important for the child to perceive the world, their education and social interactions. An infant who appears not to see well may have **delayed visual maturation** or a more serious cause. Measuring visual acuity in children requires skill and patience, but even simple techniques can be used to elicit vision and reassure the parent.

Newborn child up to 2 months

Assessment of vision in the neonate is dependant on the age and behavioural state of the child. Because the child is pre-verbal you depend on their eye movements for information about visual function. If the child is smiling (usually at 6 weeks), then you smile at the child without making any noise, and if they smile back, you know they can see!

There are a number of techniques used to test vision.

Fix and follow

• Use a large brightly coloured shiny toy to see if the child fixes and follows.

• With the child sitting on their mother's knee, move the toy *slowly* from left to right about 50 cm in front of the child's face. If the child can see he will only follow the toy if he is awake and if the toy is moved extremely slowly as eye movements are immature at this age.

• If possible, test each eye separately, by occluding one eye with an occlusive patch.

• If the child fixes and follows the target, record the vision as '**fixes and follows**'.

• If the child doesn't follow the toy this may be because he can't see or is drowsy, or he is just not interested—try again later.

Spinning

Whilst **spinning** the child, observe his eye movements. He will have nystagmus during spinning if he can see. This is the vestibulo-ocular reflex or VOR. When you stop, the nystagmus will change direction for 1 or 2 beats in a seeing child. This is post-rotational nystagmus. If it persists the child is either severely visually impaired or has a cortical lesion.

Other clinical tests

Preferential looking (PL) and visual evoked potentials (VEP).

• PL: a card with different sized grating patterns on one side and plain on the other is shown to the infant who will look towards the grating side if they can see it.

• VEP: the child has electrodes on its head which record brain signals if they see the pattern on the screen.

Infant (up to 2 years)
Cardiff cards

• A more accurate way of recording vision in these infants is to use **Cardiff cards** (CC).

• Each card has a line drawing of a familiar object on either the upper or lower half of the card, and the thickness of the lines vary. According to the thickness of the line, the card will have a letter (e.g. CC H) and a Snellen equivalent (Sn Eq) on the back (e.g. 6/6 for the finest line).

• From a distance of 50 cm or 1 m, the cards are rapidly shown to the child and the examiner observes the child making vertical eye movements up and down to the corresponding picture, and records the acuity as, for example, 'CC H at 50 cm–Sn Eq 6/9'. If possible the acuity of each eye should be recorded separately.

Toddler (2–3 years)

Once the child can speak you can ask them to identify verbally some simple and familiar pictures.

Kay's pictures

• The most common method of assessing vision in this group is with Kay's pictures. This test consists of a booklet of cards, on each of which there is a line drawing.

• Each line drawing has a Snellen equivalent depending on the size of the drawing (i.e. the largest drawing is equivalent to the 6/60 letter on the Snellen chart).

• The examiner stands 6 m from the child and asks him to identify each picture.

• If the child is too shy to tell you what each picture is he will usually whisper it to his parent who in turn will indicate to you if he was correct.

Young children (4–5 years)
Sheridan–Gardner test

• The child is given a card with several letters randomly arranged on it.

• The examiner stands 6 m away and presents single letters on a card of varying Snellen equivalence.

• The child is asked to match each letter with the letter on his card. Each eye is examined separately and the acuity recorded.

KEY POINTS

• In newborn children use 'fix and follow' or spinning to elicit presence of vision.
• In infant less than 2 years old use Cardiff cards.
• In infants aged 2–3 years use Kay's pictures.
• In children aged 4–5 years use Sheridan–Gardner letters.

21 Strabismus (squints)

Examination

Corneal Hirschberg reflection test – to detect a squint
- ☐ The **corneal reflex** position is observed – each mm of displacement is equal to about 15 prism dioptres (7 degrees)

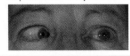

Example: Right 45 prism dioptre convergent squint (esotropia)

The cover tests

1. The cover–uncover test – to detect the presence of a squint:
- ☐ Observe if one eye is preferred for fixation
- ☐ Ask the patient to look at the fixation target – if in a child this can be a light or toy
- ☐ Occlude (for a few seconds) the eye that appears to be fixing. As you cover the eye, watch the other uncovered eye to see if it moves to take up fixation
- ☐ Remove the occluder and see if the original eye retakes up fixation. If it does, it is the preferred fixating eye and the other eye has a squint (non-alternating heterotropia)
- ☐ Do this for near and then distance vision

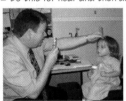

2. The alternate cover test – to detect a latent squint or phoria in a patient with straight eyes on cover test:
- ☐ Ask the patient to fixate on an object
- ☐ Cover one eye then rapidly move cover to the other eye
- ☐ Repeat rapidly several times
- ☐ Observe the movement of the covered eye as it becomes uncovered
- ☐ If it moves inwards to take up fixation the patient has an 'exophoria'
- ☐ Do test for near and then distance

Also can be used with a prism bar to measure the maximum size of a squint

- -

Example cover test:
When the left fixing eye is covered with an opaque occluder, the right eye moves inwards to take up fixation of the target. The squint is divergent (exotropia)

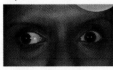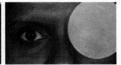

Squint

The size of the squint is measured with a prism bar

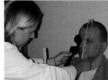

Prism alternate cover test

Long-sight (hypermetropia) and convergent squint (esotropia)

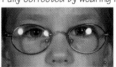   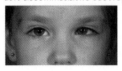

Left accommodative esotropia   Fully corrected by wearing hypermetropic glasses

Assessment of ocular movements in 9 positions of gaze (primary gaze and 8 directions)

Note the defective movement of the left eye in left gaze in left lateral rectus palsy

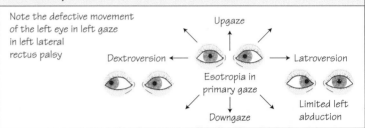

Upgaze

Dextroversion ← → Latroversion

Esotropia in primary gaze

Downgaze

Limited left abduction

Amblyopia therapy - Patching

Left good eye is patched in order to encourage use of right amblyopic eye

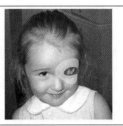

Orthoptic definitions

- ■ **i) Strabismus / squint**
  Malalignment of the two eyes. If it is constantly present, it is manifest, but if it is only detected on dissociation with an alternate cover–uncover test, it is latent
- ■ **ii) Binocular single vision (BSV)**
  The use of both eyes together to achieve binocular depth perception – stereopsis
- ■ **iii) Amblyopia – 'lazy eye' in 2% of the population**
  Amblyopia occurs from insufficient use of the eye(s) during visual development (birth – 7 years) commonly due to the presence of a manifest squint and/or refractive error. The brain suppresses the image from a deviating or defocused eye, particularly under 2 years of age – the sensitive period – when visual development is especially vulnerable to disruption. Other causes include congenital cataract or ptosis
- ■ **iv) Amblyopia therapy**
  The treatment of squints in childhood with glasses and patching
- ■ **v) Heterophoria = latent strabismus**
  Both eyes look straight but deviate on dissociation. It is common and usually does not need treatment. Types: esophoria – convergent (inwards), exophoria – divergent (outwards), hyperphoria – upward, hypophoria – downward
- ■ **vi) Heterotropia = manifest strabismus in 5 – 8% of the population**
  One or other eye is not directed towards the fixation point. Types: esotropia – convergent, exotropia – divergent, hypertropia – upward, hypotropia – downward
- ■ **vii) Concomitant strabismus**
  The deviation remains the same in all directions of gaze
- ■ **viii) Incomitant strabismus**
  The angle of deviation changes with the direction of gaze
- ■ **ix) Patching**
  The patch completely covers the good eye to encourage the bad eye (amblyopic one) to be used and develop vision. Generally unsuccessful after age 7 years
- ■ **x) Diplopia**
  Double vision

Aims

1 Understand squint terminology.
2 Do a cover test to detect a squint.
3 Know the basic principles of amblyopia therapy.

Children with a squint will not 'grow out' of it. There may be a sinister cause such as cataract or retinoblastoma, so do a red reflex. Any child suspected of having a squint should be referred to an orthoptist and ophthalmologist for assessment.

Orthoptists are allied health professionals who assess patients with diplopia, strabismus and eye movement defects. They work closely with **ophthalmologists** in the management of children's visual development, testing paediatric visual acuity (see Chapter 20) and treating amblyopia.

Aetiology and pathophysiology

Concomitant strabismus

- Binocular single vision (BSV) usually develops by 3–5 months old. If BSV does not 'lock in', esotropia (convergent squint) can develop at this time, although most concomitant squints develop later at around 2–4 years, particularly with hypermetropia.
- Any cause of reduced vision in one eye interrupts BSV and results in a squint, e.g. cataract, retinoblastoma or anisometropia.
- Children with a family history of strabismus or refractive error and those with developmental abnormalities have a higher incidence of concomitant squint.

Incomitant strabismus

- Congenital causes are rare, e.g. third, fourth or sixth nerve palsy.
- Acquired incomitant squint presents with diplopia in adults. A child may adopt a compensatory head posture to minimize diplopia and therefore may not complain of diplopia. A very young child will suppress the second image and develop amblyopia if untreated.
- Acquired causes include cranial nerve palsy (paralytic) secondary to intracranial pathology, thyroid eye disease and postorbital floor fracture (restrictive).

Management

Orthoptists, optometrists and ophthalmologists collaborate in the management of squint using a combination of glasses, surgery and orthoptic treatment.

Childhood concomitant and congenital incomitant squint

Orthoptist

- Measures visual acuity (VA).
- Detects and measures squint using cover tests.
- Assesses eye movements.
- Assesses binocular vision (including tests for stereopsis).
- Monitors amblyopia therapy with patching ± atropine occlusion.

Refraction

The optometrist or ophthalmologist performs refraction (cycloplegic if child aged <7 years). In fully or partial accommodative esotropia with high hypermetropia, wearing glasses will fully or partially correct the squint as well as improve visual acuity, and surgery may not be required.

Amblyopia therapy

Spectacles (if applicable) and a patch worn on the better eye for a specified number of hours per day, depending on the child's age and VA.

Surgery

Strabismus surgery is performed if the squint is socially unacceptable and to restore/improve binocular vision. In esotropia, the horizontal rectus muscles are operated; recessing the medial rectus and resecting the lateral rectus or bimedial rectus recessions.

Acquired incomitant squint (children and adults)

- The underlying cause must be established and treated (e.g. intracranial tumour, diabetes, hypertension).
- Orthoptic management is by joining diplopia with Fresnel prisms or prisms incorporated into the spectacle prescription.
- Surgery is performed if BSV is not comfortably restored once the extraocular muscle(s) recover or have been stable for at least 6 months.

KEY POINTS

- Esotropia is a convergent squint.
- Amblyopia must be treated *early — ideally before age 5 years*.
- Beware: squint may be a presentation of an intracranial tumour or retinoblastoma.

Leukokoria

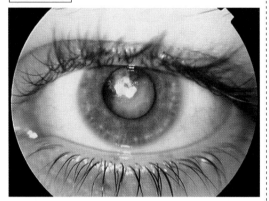

Leukokoria – a white coloured pupil – exclude congenital cataract or retinoblastoma

Retinoblastoma

Hereditary (usually bilateral) or sporadic (usually unilateral)

Treatment: Radioactive plaque or enucleation and adjuvant chemotherapy

Survival: Untreated only 2–4 years (brain metastases). Treated 90–95% 5 year survival

Retinopathy of prematurity

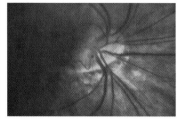

Dragged disc

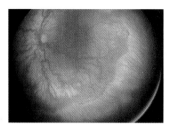

Proliferating retinal vessels on ridge

There is an International classification of retinopathy of prematurity (ROP) where worsening stages are recognized. The retina is divided into zones for its development

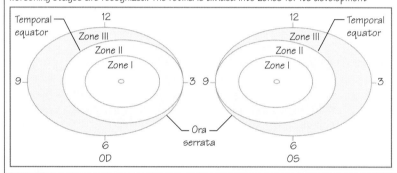

Screening for ROP

- Infants <1500 g
- 31 weeks or less gestational age
- Begin at 6 weeks post-natally, not immediately
- Two-weekly intervals
- Weekly if ROP develops until it regresses or is treated
- Indirect ophthalmoscopy and indenter to see the peripheral retina (pupils dilated)

Congenital glaucoma with buphthalmos

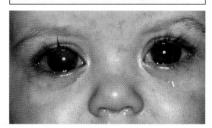

Buphthalmos—child with big watering photophobic eyes and corneal oedema

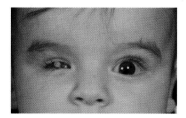

Buphthalmos examination under anaesthesia— intra-ocular pressure monitoring with hand-held tonometer

CNLDO

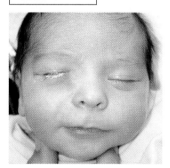

Congenital nasolacrimal duct obstruction

Microphthalmia

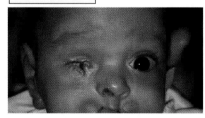

Right eyelid coloboma and microphthalmos. Partial cryptophthalmus (hidden eye)

Right microphthalmia with soft tissue expander. Left iris coloboma

Aims

1 Differential diagnosis of leukokoria.
2 Main sight-threatening eye problems in neonates.
3 Management of a watering eye.

In a neonate the three most important topics are leukokoria, retinoblastoma and ophthalmia neonatorum.

Leukokoria

A white-coloured pupillary reflex seen when an ophthalmoscope is shone at the pupil. Causes include:
- Congenital cataract.
- Hyperplastic primary persistant vitreous (HPPV).
- Retinoblastoma.
- Infections: toxoplasmosis and toxocariasis.
- Retinopathy of prematurity (ROP).
- Coats' disease.

Congenital cataract

- Presents as leukokoria, a dull red reflex, squint or nystagmus.
- If bilateral, the child may be visually inattentive.
- The eye may be smaller but there is usually no relative afferent papillary defect unless there is other retinal or optic nerve pathology.
- Causes include: idiopathic (most common), familial autosomal dominant, galactosaemia and rubella (also causes microcephaly, congenital heart defects, corneal clouding and retinopathy).
- Needs *urgent* (within days) assessment with a view to cataract surgery and subsequent amblyopia therapy. Some cataracts are small and need monitoring and amblyopia therapy.

Retinoblastoma

- This malignant tumour of the retina is the most common intraocular tumour of childhood.
- It often appears as a white mass growing into the vitreous and causing leukokoria when it is advanced/big.
- Urgent assessment and treatment is required by a joint paediatric oncology and paediatric ophthalmology team in a specialist centre.

Non-accidental injury (NAI)

A neonate with leukokoria or ocular trauma may have NAI.

Retinopathy of prematurity (ROP)

- This important cause of childhood blindness occurs in pre-term babies and is screened for by ophthalmologists.
- Treatment with cryotherapy or laser has limited success in threshold disease.
- Prevention remains the key.
- Advanced/untreated ROP may have leukokoria.
- Complications of treatment include cataract and myopia.
- In severe ROP with retinal detachment, vitreoretinal surgery is often only palliative.

Ophthalmia neonatorum

- Notifiable disease.
- The neonate usually has a unilateral or bilateral purulent conjunctivitis within a few days of birth.
- The ophthalmologist must examine the child and take swabs/scrapes for bacteria (including Gram and Giemsa stains), *Chlamydia* immunofluorescent antibody test and viral culture.

- Suspect *Neisseria gonorrhoeae* or *Chlamydia trachomatis* until proved otherwise as both can cause blindness.
- Systemic and topical treatment is essential.
- Refer both parents to STD clinic.

Buphthalmos (see Chapter 36)

- A large eye in an infant associated with congenital glaucoma and a cause of blindness/defective vision.
- The infant has photosensitivity and watering with elevated intraocular pressure.
- Needs specialized paediatric ophthalmology management.

Anophthalmos and microphthalmos

- Rare total absence of an eye (anophthalmos) or a very small ocular remnant (microphthalmos).
- The aim of management is to promote orbital bony development by keeping the ocular remnant (microphthalmos or cyst) and expanding the soft tissue of the orbit and eyelids sequentially, prior to placing an ocular prosthesis (artificial eye).

Watering eyes/epiphora due to congenital nasolacrimal duct obstruction (NLDO)

- Causes watery sticky eyes.
- Aetiology: opening of the lower end of the nasolacrimal duct (where it enters the nose in the inferior meatus at the valve of Hasner) is often delayed for several months. Rare causes include absent canaliculus and absent or imperforate punctum.
- Treatment of congenital NLDO:
  —Advise the parent that the watering is likely to resolve by age 1 year in 90%.
  —Daily small finger massage over the lacrimal sac at the medial canthus to open the valve.
  —Clean the eyelids with sterile saline.
  —Antibiotic drops are only rarely required.
  —If there is an amniocoele (bluish lump) it will usually resolve with systemic antibiotic course. If this doesn't work do an early probing at <2 month's age.
  —An expressible mucocoele suggests nasolacrimal duct block requiring dacryocystorhinostomy surgery.
  —For persistant watering aged over 1 year, do a syringe and probing (S&P) ± nasal endoscopic monitering.
  —If recurrent epiphora, repeat S&P with endoscopic monitoring and consider intubation or dacryocystorhinostomy (DCR).

Ptosis (see Chapter 23)

A neonate with an upper eyelid drooping across the visual axis should be referred urgently to an ophthalmologist with a view to urgent frontalis suspension surgery and amblyopia therapy. Otherwise usually wait until age 4 years if visual development is not threatened.

KEY POINTS
- Leukokoria—retinoblastoma and congenital cataract.
- A watering eye from congenital NLDO usually resolves by 1 year.
- Beware: congenital glaucoma may present with large or watery eyes.

Differential diagnosis in orbital cellulitis

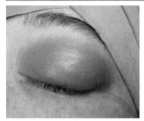

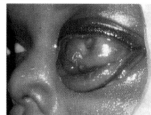

- Rare malignant orbital tumour of childhood that can metastasize. It may present as orbital cellulitis
- Average age of onset: 7 years
- Grows fast and progresses
- If suspected, urgent referral and biopsy required

Post-septal orbital cellulitis – pre-drainage

Rhabdomyosarcoma

Infants and older children

The most common visual problems (apart from myopia) have usually been detected by age 2–4 years. The problems of a child over 2 and under 12 years relate commonly to the eyelids, lacrimal system and orbits. Teenagers have their own visual problems with the onset of myopia, presentation of Leber's optic neuropathy (usually in mid to late teens), "hysterical" loss of vision, headaches and convergence insufficiency. Reduced vision from albinism has usually been detected by this age

Ptosis

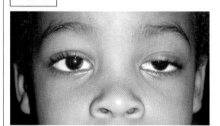

Congenital left ptosis

Allergy

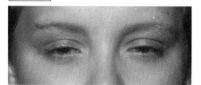

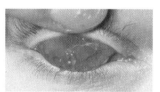

Vernal keratoconjunctivitis causing bilateral acquired ptosis

Vernal giant papillae

Lumps on and around eyelid

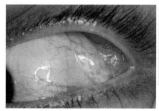

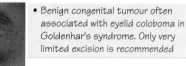

- Benign congenital conjunctival and subconjunctival yellow fatty lesion. Lies very close to the lacrimal ductules, therefore excision is not advised as it risks a severe dry eye from lacrimal ductile damage

Orbital, peri-orbital and eyelid haemangioma

Dermolipoma

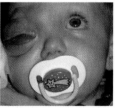

- Benign congenital tumour often associated with eyelid coloboma in Goldenhar's syndrome. Only very limited excision is recommended

Limbal dermoid

 Dermoid cyst

- Smooth round non-tender relatively immobile lump in the superolateral > superomedial orbit that gradually grows in size. Risk of rupture if in a prominent position. CT scan is required to assess extent and plan surgery. Removal of an intact cyst is necessary as its yellow cheesy contents are very irritant

Infections

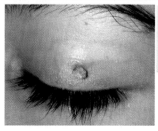

- Endemic in schools
- Causes chronic follicular conjunctivitis. Small dome-shaped itchy lesions around the eyelids and on the hands or arms

Molluscum contagiosum

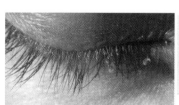

- Typically from pubic lice – unilateral or bilateral causing itchy eyes with crusty lashes from the nits and blood-tinged debris. Pilocarpine gel to remove

Headlice = pediculosis

Aims

1 Identify common paediatric eyelid and orbital problems.
2 Know why and when to operate on ptosis.
3 Management of orbital cellulitis.

The infant has different problems from the neonate. The most important condition is orbital cellulitis, which must be diagnosed and treated promptly. Other common paediatric problems encountered include persistent mild drooping eyelid (ptosis), a sticky watering eye and eyelid lumps.

Squints are covered in Chapter 21.

Orbital cellulitis

Distinguish between pre-septal and post-septal orbital cellulitis. The child can be quite ill and febrile, and requires admission.

Pre-septal

- Pre-septal involves only the eyelids but can spread posterior to the orbital septum to become post-septal.
- One or both eyelids are swollen and tender.
- White eye, which moves fully with no impairment of vision or proptosis.
- Treat with i.v. antibiotics.

Post-septal

- Potentially severe life-threatening condition (cavernous sinus thrombosis), unless treated.
- Painful orbital/eyelid red swelling and proptosis; child is feverish and unwell.
- Associated with an upper respiratory tract infection and undiagnosed sinusitis.
- May not be able to open eye to see limited eye movements.
- Conjunctiva red and swollen.
- Vision may be affected: reduced visual acuity and red desaturation with a relative afferent papillary defect due to optic nerve compression.
- Do a CT scan to exclude sinus disease and subperiosteal abscess, which need surgical draining and bacteriology.
- Infection from: *Haemophilus infuenzae*, *Streptococcus*, *Staphylococcus negative rods* or *Gram*.
- Urgent admission, blood cultures and treatment with i.v. antibiotics.

> **WARNING**
> Rhabdomyosarcoma and leukaemia are important differential diagnoses of bacterial orbital cellulitis.

Ptosis (drooping eyelid)

- Congenital dystrophic.
- Acquired third cranial nerve palsy (rare).
- Inflammation, e.g. vernal keratoconjunctivitis.

Ptosis assessment

Measure the visual acuity, strength of the levator muscle in millimetres (**levator function**), vertical palpebral aperture distance and skin crease height. Observe Bell's phenomenon. Look for aberrant eyelid movements with chewing and talking to detect Marcus Gunn jaw–winking ptosis. Check under the eyelid.

Type of surgery

This depends largely on the level of the levator function. If the levator function is very poor (<5 mm) the eyelid is internally suspended to the frontalis muscle (frontalis suspension). If there is good levator function, the levator muscle is shortened (anterior levator resection, ALR). When there is a risk of amblyopia in neonate because the lid covers the pupil most of the time, then urgent frontalis suspension with a prolene suture is required.

The child may later need autogenous fascia lata frontalis suspension (where fascial strips are taken from their upper leg).

If the eyelid is only slightly drooping and the child can easily 'see out from beneath it' by adopting a small chin-up head position, there is less risk of amblyopia and the child can wait until aged 4 years before having ptosis surgery.

> **Persistant sticky watering eyes**
> - Blocked nasolacrimal duct requires dacryocystorhinostomy (DCR).
> - Vernal/atopic conjunctivitis. Photophobic with swollen eyelids and itchy, stringy discharge that is worse in summer—can give an acquired ptosis. History of atopy. Large giant papillae on tarsal conjunctiva and possibly small limbal lumps (limbal vernal). Treat with topical anti-inflammatory drops.
> - Blepharitis. Red rimmed sticky eyes with a tendency to recurrent blepharoconjunctivitis and watering. Treat with lid toilet and topical antibiotic ointment.

Lumps on and around the eye

There are many different lumps—identify capillary haemangioma, dermolipoma, limbal dermoid and dermoid cyst.

Capillary haemangioma

Swelling appears at birth or shortly afterwards, then increases in size for about 6 months. Most common in the superonasal orbit and eyelid. Grows slowly, during which it can cause mechanical ptosis and risk of amblyopia if the lid covers the visual axis or its weight causes astigmatism. Treated with local infiltration of steroids to speed up resolution and reduce the bulk of the haemangioma. Spontaneously regresses usually after age 1 year.

Stye (external hordeolum)

- Lash follicle infection—hot red lump that resolves rapily.

Chalazion

- Lump due to an inflamed blocked meibomian gland duct, which will usually gradually resolve over a few weeks without treatment.
- Topical antibiotic ointment for 7–10 days.
- Incise and curette under short general anaesthetic if not improving with treatment (see Chapter 24).

KEY POINTS
- Ptosis—risk of amblyopia when eyelid covers the visual axis.
- Ptosis—usually wait until age 4 years before surgery is done.
- Drain subperiosteal abscess in orbital cellulitis.

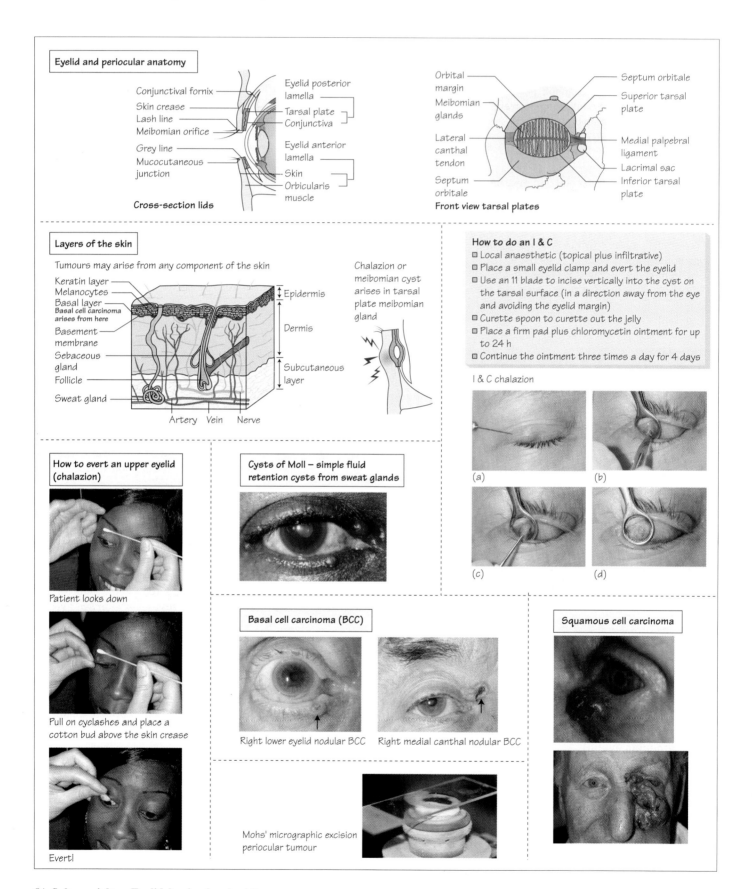

Eyelid and periocular anatomy

Conjunctival fornix
Skin crease
Lash line
Meibomian orifice
Grey line
Mucocutaneous junction

Eyelid posterior lamella
Tarsal plate
Conjunctiva
Eyelid anterior lamella
Skin
Orbicularis muscle

Cross-section lids

Orbital margin
Meibomian glands
Lateral canthal tendon
Septum orbitale

Septum orbitale
Superior tarsal plate
Medial palpebral ligament
Lacrimal sac
Inferior tarsal plate

Front view tarsal plates

Layers of the skin

Tumours may arise from any component of the skin

Keratin layer
Melanocytes
Basal layer
Basal cell carcinoma arises from here
Basement membrane
Sebaceous gland
Follicle
Sweat gland

Epidermis
Dermis
Subcutaneous layer

Artery Vein Nerve

Chalazion or meibomian cyst arises in tarsal plate meibomian gland

How to do an I & C
- Local anaesthetic (topical plus infiltrative)
- Place a small eyelid clamp and evert the eyelid
- Use an 11 blade to incise vertically into the cyst on the tarsal surface (in a direction away from the eye and avoiding the eyelid margin)
- Curette spoon to curette out the jelly
- Place a firm pad plus chloromycetin ointment for up to 24 h
- Continue the ointment three times a day for 4 days

I & C chalazion

(a)　　　(b)
(c)　　　(d)

How to evert an upper eyelid (chalazion)

Patient looks down

Pull on eyelashes and place a cotton bud above the skin crease

Evert!

Cysts of Moll – simple fluid retention cysts from sweat glands

Basal cell carcinoma (BCC)

Right lower eyelid nodular BCC　　Right medial canthal nodular BCC

Mohs' micrographic excision periocular tumour

Squamous cell carcinoma

Aims

1 Recognize a chalazion and understand its treatment.
2 Recognize a basal cell carcinoma.
3 Treatment of periocular basal cell carcinoma.

Differential diagnosis of periocular tumours

Many different lumps are found on the eyelids, both benign and malignant.

- Benign: chalazion, papilloma, retention cyst and sebaceous cyst.
- Malignant:
  —basal cell carcinoma (BCC);
  —squamous cell carcinoma (SCC);
  —sebaceous gland carcinoma (SGC);
  —malignant melanoma;
  —Merkel cell tumour;
  —other rare, e.g. sweat gland tumours.

Benign lumps

Chalazion/meibomian cyst

Inflamed painful lid swelling due to a blocked meibomian duct—there are at least 27 ducts in each eyelid and each one has the potential to block! Initial treatment in an adult is by hot compresses and topical antibiotic ointment four times a day for 2 weeks. If the lump persists, do an incision and curettage (I&C).

If an assumed chalazion recurs, particularly in an older person, do an incisional biopsy urgently for histopathological analysis as this may be a **sebaceous gland carcinoma (meibomian gland carcinoma)**. *This is highly malignant.*

Solar keratoses (actinic keratoses)

These are dry scaly patches due to dysplastic intraepidermal proliferation of atypical keratinocytes and occur on the face in older, fair-skinned persons who have lived in sunny climates. There is a low risk of malignant transformation into squamous cell carcinoma. Fortunately many solar keratoses regress spontaneously over 1–2 years, but 15% recur. Treatment is with cryotherapy or 5-fluorouracil.

Malignant lumps

Basal cell carcinoma ('Rodent ulcer')

This is the commonest periocular malignant tumour. It occurs most commonly on the lower eyelid, then medial canthus, upper lid and lateral canthus. It is typically a nodular pearly lump with no hair or lashes on it, but with telangiectatic blood vessels. The central zone may bleed and ulcerate. It can be morphoeic and have indistinct margins. It grows slowly by direct extension and destroys tissue locally. It can invade the orbit if neglected or inadequately treated. Early treatment is recommended—incisional biopsy to make the diagnosis and excisional biopsy with a 2–4 mm margin of clear tissue, to completely remove the tumour.

Nodular BCC is the commonest form and its edges are easy to define. There is a rarer morphoeic type with ill-defined edges and extent, which is more difficult to manage and has a higher recurrence rate. BCC does not metastasize. Surgical excision and reconstruction is the mainstay of treatment of BCC although cryotherapy and radiotherapy are occasional options.

Mohs' micrographic surgery

Mohs' micrographic excision of BCC is a special technique to remove the tumour with frozen sections of the deep bed of the tumour to ensure complete excision, done by dermatological surgeons especially trained in the technique. It provides good clearance of tumour with maximum normal tissue preservation and low recurrence. An oculoplastics-trained ophthalmologist then does the periocular reconstruction.

Squamous cell carcinoma

SCC is rarer than BCC but more rapidly growing with a greater potential for spread, especially perineural. It is a red lump with a variable appearance. It is much more common in immunosuppressed patients, for instance post renal or liver transplant patients on long-term immunosuppression drugs.

Sebaceous gland carcinoma

SGC may masquerade as a recurrent chalazion or unilateral blepharitis in an elderly female patient. A large incisional biopsy is required for histopathologic analysis. This tumour can spread by lymphatics and the patient requires radical neck excision. There is a significant 5-year mortality.

Malignant melanoma

Very rare but potentially very serious. Most pigmented lesions around the eye are benign but the usual caveats apply—if there is an increase in size or bleeds, urgent referral is needed.

KEY POINTS

- A recurrent chalazion may be a malignant tumour—sebaceous gland carcinoma.
- Basal cell carcinoma is the commonest eyelid malignancy.
- Mohs' micrographic surgery is the gold standard for excising periocular basal cell carcinoma.

25 Common eyelid malpositions

Nerve supply to eyelids
Upper eyelid
Levator palpebrae superioris (cranial nerve III) and Müller's superior tarsal muscle (sympathetic) open the upper eyelid
Orbicularis oculi (cranial nerve VII) closes the eyelid
Lower eyelid
The capsulopalpebral fascia (linked to the inferior rectus muscle – cranial nerve III) and Müller's lower tarsal muscle (sympathetic) help the lower lid move 2–4 mm downwards on downgaze and help open the lids
Orbicularis oculi (cranial nerve VII) closes the eyelid

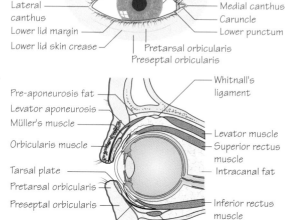

Supracilia, Upper lid skin fold, Cilia, Lateral canthus, Lower lid margin, Lower lid skin crease, Limbus, Upper punctum, Plica, Medial canthus, Caruncle, Lower punctum, Pretarsal orbicularis, Preseptal orbicularis

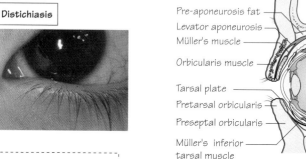

Pre-aponeurosis fat, Levator aponeurosis, Müller's muscle, Orbicularis muscle, Tarsal plate, Pretarsal orbicularis, Preseptal orbicularis, Müller's inferior tarsal muscle, Whitnall's ligament, Levator muscle, Superior rectus muscle, Intracanal fat, Inferior rectus muscle, Inferior oblique muscle

Entropion

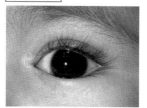

Congenital lower lid entropion – epiblepharon

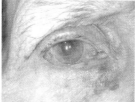 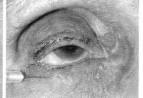

Involutional lower lid entropion
i) Causing red sore eye

ii) Botulinum toxin A temporary oricularis chemodenervation (surgery is the definitive treatment)

Distichiasis

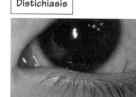

Ectropion

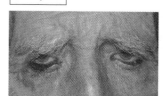 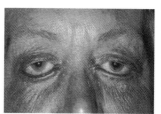

Involutional ectropion

Cicatricial ectropion
Contact dermatitis from glaucoma drops (reversible on stopping drops)

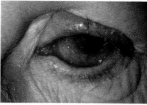 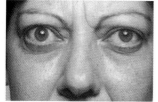

Facial palsy with anaesthtic cornea (VIIth and Vth CN palsies) causing neurotrophic keratitis and scarring

Graves' orbitopathy (thyroid eye disease) – mild proptosis, right upper and bilateral lower lid retraction

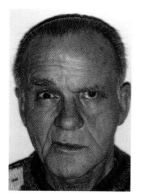

Facial palsy (lower motor neurone) and lagophthalmos

Eyelid and brow measurements

LidF, UMRD, LMRD, LSS, ULB, PA

ULB = Upper lid brow
PA = Palpebral aperture
LidF = Lid fold
UMRD = Upper margin reflex distance
LMRD = Lower margin reflex distance
LSS = Lower scleral show

Lateral tarsal strip

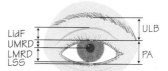

Used to shorten eyelid in entropion and ectropion surgery

The lateral tarsal strip is tucked into the lateral orbit at the lateral canthus and sutured to the periosteum at the lateral orbital rim. This is a widely used useful technique

Definitions	
Trichiasis	= rubbing of abnormal inturned eyelashes against the eye causing discomfort
Distichiasis	= additional row of aberrant lashes arising from the meibomian orifices

Aims

1 Examine an eyelid.
2 Identify entropion (lid in) and ectropion (lid out).
3 Identify ptosis (lid down) and eyelid retraction (lid up).

Lid function

- Ocular protection.
- Tear film distribution.

> **Examine an eyelid**
> - Measure visual acuity!
> - Look at the whole face, eyebrow height and symmetry
> - Measure the vertical palpebral aperture (PA) and margin reflex distances (MRDs) and amount of scleral show (SS) above or below the limbus in mm
> - Measure the levator function (LF) in mm—upperlid excursion from full downgaze to full upgaze
> - Assess orbicularis strength and Bell's phenomenon (do the eyes roll upwards under lid on closure?)
> - Exclude aberrant movements
> - Lag on downgaze—eyelid hangs up a bit on downgaze
> - Detect lagophthalmos—eye remains partially open on attempted closure
> - Exclude distichiasis, trichiasis, entropion and ectropion
> - Examine tarsal conjunctiva and conjunctival fornices to exclude scar or tumour

Entropion

Entropion: Eyelid turns in towards cornea and lashes touch the surface of the eye.

Aetiology
- Involutional—older persons.
- Spastic (causes by severe squeezing of the eyelids in response to ocular discomfort).
- Cicatricial entropion secondary to conjunctival scarring, e.g. staphylococcal lid margin disease (mild entropion) or ocular cicatricial pemphigoid (severe entropion) or trachoma.

Pathogenesis
Thinning of the lamellae and disinsertion of the lower lid retractors. The pre-septal overrides the pretarsal orbicularis causing inturning of the lower lid.

Symptoms
Ocular irritation, discomfort, reflex watering (hypersecretion), redness and occasionally keratitis if left untreated. It is worse lying down, e.g. reading in bed.

Treatment
1 Temporary treatment:
- Lid taping and topical lubricants.
- Botulinum toxin A injected into the pre-septal orbicularis alleviates symptoms for up to 4 months but has to be repeated.
2 Surgery is the mainstay of treatment.
- Lateral tarsal strip with everting sutures (LTS + ES). This shortens the lower eyelid horizontally and everts the eyelid.
- Simple everting sutures (ES) alone.

Ectropion

Ectropion: Lower eyelid turns outwards away from the eye.

Aetiology
- Involutional—older persons.
- Cicatricial causes, e.g. post blepharoplasty, actinic, following skin tumour excision, etc., and contact dermatitis.
- Mechanical—the weight of an eyelid tumour pulling the eyelid outwards.
- Facial palsy (VIIth nerve palsy).

Symptoms
Watering, irritation, grittiness and redness.

Treatment
- Involutional ectropion—shorten the eyelid horizontally and turn the medial part inwards using a lateral tarsal strip and excision of a diamond shape of medial tarsal conjunctiva or medial spindle (LTS + MS).
- Cicatricial ectropion—skin graft or flap to lengthen the anterior lamella; horizontal shortening may also be required.
- Contact dermatitis—stop the causative eye drops or change to preservative-free drops. No surgery needed.
- For facial palsy, see below.

Ptosis

Definition of eyelid ptosis: Abnormally low position of the upper eyelid margin caused by poor function of the levator palpebrae superioris or Müller's muscle.

Paediatric ptosis see Chapter 23.
Aetiology:
- Involutional or aponeurotic (thinning or dehiscence of the anterior part of the levator, the aponeurosis). There is good levator function (LF). Occurs commonly in the elderly.
- Myogenic. LF is very poor. Includes the congenital dystrophic (fatty) levator muscles in children and myopathies in adults, e.g. chronic progressive external ophthalmoplegia.
- Neurogenic. The LF is usually poor, e.g. IIIrd nerve palsy.
- Mechanical. Usually good LF. A tumour weighs the eyelid down, e.g. neurofibromatosis.
- Traumatic ptosis may be aponeurotic, myogenic or neurogenic.

Symptoms
- Cosmetically poor appearance.
- Functional—reduces the visual field.

Management
Depends on the type of ptosis and LF. Normal or good LF is >10 mm. Moderate LF is 5–10 mm. Poor LF is <5 mm.
- Good and moderate LF: anterior levator resection—tuck / advance the levator aponeurosis or muscle.
- Poor LF: frontalis suspension with autogenous fascia lata.

Eyelid retraction

Lower motor neurone facial palsy (7th CN palsy) and thyroid eye disease can both cause exposure keratitis. See Chapters 28 and 49.

> **KEY POINTS**
> - Measurement is important in eyelids.
> - Involutional entropion is treated temporarily with botulinum toxin A.
> - Facial palsy causes lagophthalmos and a risk of exposure keratitis.

Lacrimal anatomy
The lacrimal drainage system consists of the punta, canaliculi, lacrimal sac and nasolacrimal duct (NLD)

Lacrimal physiology
The tears are produced by the lacrimal gland and the accessory lacrimal tissue (glands of Krause and Wolfring) and are swept over the eye surface with each blink. Tear evaporation occurs (approximately 25%). The marginal tear strip drains via the lower canaliculus predominantly (70%) and 30% via the upper canaliculus. The lacrimal pump mechanism refers to the action of the eyelids contracting and pumping the tears into the lacrimal sac

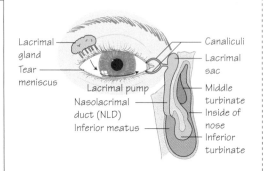

Lacrimal gland
Tear meniscus
Lacrimal pump
Nasolacrimal duct (NLD)
Inferior meatus
Canaliculi
Lacrimal sac
Middle turbinate
Inside of nose
Inferior turbinate

Lacrimal syringing

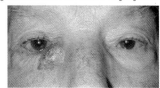

Nasal endoscopy
This is a very useful technique that provides direct observation of the nasal space both in out-patients and during lacrimal surgery. A rigid Hopkins 4 mm 0° rigid nasal endoscope is used to look at the opening of the NLD into the nose and at the DCR surgery site

Right mucocoele–chronic dacryocystitis

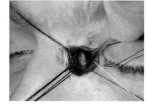

Normal dacryocystography (DCG) – left side shows free drainage contrast media into nose

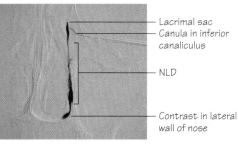

Lacrimal sac
Canula in inferior canaliculus
NLD
Contrast in lateral wall of nose

DCG shows right anatomically blocked NLD. Note that no contrast material is seen entering the NLD

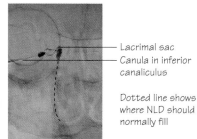

Lacrimal sac
Canula in inferior canaliculus
Dotted line shows where NLD should normally fill

Left external skin approach dacryocystorhinostomy (DCR) – per-operative view

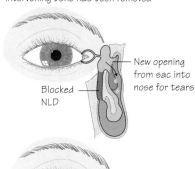

A mucosal-lined opening is made from the lacrimal sac to the nose after the intervening bone has been removed

Nuclear lacrimal scintigraphy – showing left functional NLD block

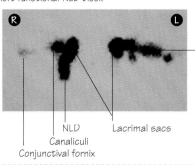

R   L

Pooling of tears containing technetium 99 in the conjunctival fornix

NLD   Lacrimal sacs
Canaliculi
Conjunctival fornix

Functioning DCR rhinostomy
Fluorescein passing freely down lateral wall of nose

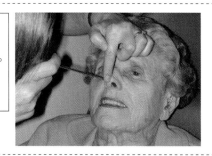

New opening from sac into nose for tears
Blocked NLD

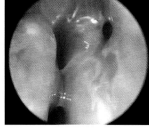

Jones Pyrex bypass tube – per-operative insertion

Endonasal endoscopic surgical DCR
– the lacrimal sac is approached from inside the nose instead of via the skin

Lacrimal sac
Keratome
Middle turbinate
Endoscope
Inferior turbinate
Floor of nose

Aims

1 Understand the difference between hypersecretion and epiphora.
2 Use of syringing in assessment of epiphora.
3 Dacryocystorhinostomy.

Nasolacrimal duct obstruction is a common cause of epiphora (watering eye). Surgery to correct this is called dacryocystorhinostomy (DCR) and can be done via the nose (endonasal) or via the skin (external). However, there are many causes of a watering eye and careful assessment is required.

Definitions

Epiphora: Reduced tear outflow from lacrimal system obstruction at any point from the punctum, canaliculus, sac and nasolacrimal duct. Nasolacrimal duct obstruction is the commonest.

Hypersecretion: Excess production of tears in response to stimulation of the trigeminal nerve from corneal irritation (e.g. corneal foreign body), dry eye or conjunctival irritation (e.g. blepharitis, conjunctivitis).

Functional epiphora: Epiphora in the presence of patent syringing without hypersecretion due to:

- eyelid malposition, e.g. lower lid ectropion;
- lacrimal pump failure, e.g. facial palsy;
- punctual, canalicular and nasolacrimal duct stenosis (without a complete obstruction).

Mucocoele: A dilated lacrimal sac containing mucous. often seen as a lump at the medial canthus. The nasolacrimal duct distal to it is blocked.

Pathogenesis

- The commonest cause of epiphora is a blocked nasolacrimal duct (NLD). This can be primary from chronic inflammation with subsequent fibrosis and stenosis, or less commonly, secondary from sarcoidosis, Wegner's, tumour or trauma. DCR is the treatment of choice.

> **WARNING**
> **Canalicular disease.** If there is severe canalicular obstruction (e.g. following radiotherapy, some chemotherapy drugs, herpes simplex infection) a DCR is done with a Jones Pyrex glass tube inserted.

Investigate the watering eye

History

Stickiness/watering worse is outside or constant. There is an inflamed or quiet lump at the medial canthus. History of nasal disease, sinusitis, polyps or nasal trauma. Previous conjunctivitis, eye drops and drugs.

Assessment of the watering eye

- External examination of the forehead, periocular and medial canthus to exclude eyelid malposition and mucocoele.
- Fluorescein dye retention test: watch a drop of fluorescein 2% rapidly disappear from the conjunctiva if the system is patent or dye retention if blocked.

- Slit lamp examination:
  —exclude blepharitis;
  —exclude punctual stenosis;
  —tear meniscus.

- *Probe and syringe/irrigate lacrimal system (use topical anaesthesia)* After the punctum has been dilated, a curved lacrimal canula is gently introduced into the canaliculus and advanced into the lacrimal sac and saline is irrigated. If there is passage of saline into the throat this indicates a patent system, whereas no passage indicates a blocked system. Sometimes only some saline goes down, indicating a partial NLD block.

- Special clinical tests: Jones' tests used to confirm and localize functional epiphora (not used much).

- Nasal endoscopy:
  —The nasal endoscope is used to look inside the nasal space preoperatively to exclude nasal pathology such as tumours, inflammation and polyps as well as anatomical variations.
  —It is also used to inspect the internal opening (rhinostomy) made by the DCR surgery and to check its function.
  —A successful DCR has a positive functional endoscopic dye test (FEDT), i.e. a drop of fluorescein 2% placed in the conjunctival fornix is seen emerging from the rhinostomy a few seconds later.

- Radiology imaging studies
  —Dacryocystography (DCG) with radio-opaque material for anatomical detail. Used to determine the site of the obstruction.
  —Lacrimal scintigraphy is a nuclear scanning technique using a drop of technetium 99 placed in the conjunctival fornix and a gamma camera to observe its passive drainage. It is used to detect physiological tear drainage in the assessment of functional NLD obstruction.

Surgery

DCR can be external (via the skin) or endonasal (via the nose).

- *Aim of DCR*. To relieve watering and/or sticky eye from NLD stenosis/obstruction by creating a functioning rhinostomy between the lacrimal sac and the nasal space.

- External (skin incision) approach DCR has the best track record and is the gold standard—success rates 95–98%.

- Endonasal DCR (via the nose) approach DCR is less invasive but also has lower results, 70–86%. The rigid nasal endoscope provides good illumination and magnification transnasally, with either: (i) laser, (ii) surgical, or (iii) powered instruments to make the rhinostomy. The xomed diamond burr has the best results.

   Many patients prefer endonasal DCR because it avoids skin incision. However, the advantage of external DCR is that its surgical outcome is still better than endonasal techniques.

KEY POINTS

- Ectropion is a cause of epiphora.
- Endoscopic endonasal DCR avoids a skin incision.
- External approach DCR still has the best results—95–98% success.

27 Basic orbital assessment

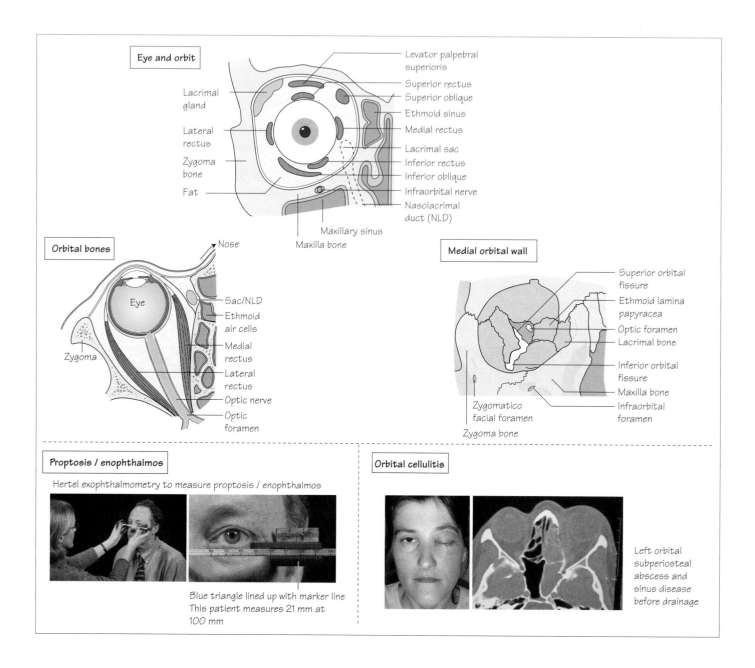

Eye and orbit
- Levator palpebral superioris
- Superior rectus
- Superior oblique
- Ethmoid sinus
- Medial rectus
- Lacrimal sac
- Inferior rectus
- Inferior oblique
- Infraorbital nerve
- Nasolacrimal duct (NLD)
- Lacrimal gland
- Lateral rectus
- Zygoma bone
- Fat
- Maxillary sinus
- Maxilla bone

Orbital bones
- Nose
- Eye
- Sac/NLD
- Ethmoid air cells
- Medial rectus
- Lateral rectus
- Optic nerve
- Optic foramen
- Zygoma

Medial orbital wall
- Superior orbital fissure
- Ethmoid lamina papyracea
- Optic foramen
- Lacrimal bone
- Inferior orbital fissure
- Maxilla bone
- Infraorbital foramen
- Zygomatico facial foramen
- Zygoma bone

Proptosis / enophthalmos

Hertel exophthalmometry to measure proptosis / enophthalmos

Blue triangle lined up with marker line
This patient measures 21 mm at 100 mm

Orbital cellulitis

Left orbital subperiosteal abscess and sinus disease before drainage

Aims

Assessment of a patient with proptosis. This chapter covers the anatomy of the orbit and the systematic approach to examining a patient with proptosis. The most common cause of proptosis in adult patients is thyroid eye disease, also known as Graves' orbitopathy.

Definitions

Proptosis: Eye protruding.
Enophthalmos: Eye sunken in.
Anophthalmia: Socket contains no eye.

Pseudophthalmia: Socket contains an orbital implant.
Microphthalmia: Socket contains a very small eye/ocular remnant.
Phthisical eye: A blind shrunken eye.
Enucleation: Removal of an eye in its entirety—detaching it from the optic nerve and the extraocular muscles.
Evisceration: Removal of the contents of the eye leaving the outer sclera, attached optic nerve and extraocular muscles.
Post-enucleation socket syndrome: Deep sunken 'eye' when the volume of the removed eye has not been adequately replaced.
Decompression orbit: Removing usually the medial and lateral orbital walls to expand the orbit in thyroid eye disease.

Orbital anatomy

The bony orbit has four margins and walls and is adjacent to the ethmoid sinus (medial) and maxillary sinus (inferior). It contains the optic foramen for the optic nerve and ophthalmic artery, the superior orbital fissure (cranial nerves and blood vessels) and inferior orbital fissure. The infraorbital nerve lies in the floor, partly in a bony canal. The orbit contains a lot of fat and connective tissue septae that support and cushion the eye and its muscles, optic nerve, nerves and blood vessels.

Orbital assessment

History

- Gradual or sudden onset. If slow/non-inflamed it is more likely to be benign.
- Unilateral or bilateral.
- Orbital swelling/sunken.
- Orbital pain.
- Periorbital redness (e.g. orbital cellulitis).
- Periorbital numbness.
- Visual disturbance.
- Double vision.
- Drooping eyelid.
- Systemic: malignancy or thyroid problem.
- Previous trauma.
- Ascultation for a bruit—caroticocavernous fistula.

Clinical examination

Visual function (if eye present) and eye examination
- Visual acuity and pupil reactions.
- Colour vision ± visual fields.
- Retina and optic disc.

Globe position
Measure **proptosis** with Hertel exophthalmometry—is it axial or non-axial?

Proptosis
- **Axial** (anteroposterior protruding globe) without horizontal or vertical displacement. This suggests a generalized orbitopathy such as thyroid eye disease or an intraconal mass.
- **Non-axial**. Horizontal or vertical displacement of globe caused by a mass pushing it sideways. For instance, a lacrimal gland tumour in the superolateral quadrant pushes the globe inferomedially.

Enophthalmos. Is there a history of trauma and possible orbital floor fracture? Is there a phthisical eye? Is there an ocular prosthesis? Has the patient had an eye enucleated? Was there an orbital implant placed after enucleation/evisceration? Is there a secondary post-enucleation socket syndrome? Are the eye movements restricted? Is the socket lining contracted?

Check cranial nerve (CN) function
- IIIrd, IVth and VIth CN: extraocular muscle movement.
- VIIth CN: upper facial musculature.
- Vth CN: corneal, periorbital and forehead sensation.

Feel the orbit
Palpate the orbital rim. If a mass is detected, is it separate from the rim? Describe its feel and shape and draw a picture of its shape and location.

Complete the examination
Palpate the temporal fossa for extension of swelling. Exclude pre-auricular, submandibular and cervical lymphadenopathy. Examine the neck for thyroid enlargement or thyroid scar. Check sensation in skin around orbit.

WARNING
Orbital tumour spread. The orbit does not have lymphatics, but extensive tumour that involves the lids and periorbital area can metastasize to local lymph nodes.

Investigations
- **CT scanning**. Axial and coronal views show the position of the optic nerve well and also the sinuses and orbital walls (request bone window settings too). Suspected vascular lesions need contrast.
- **MRI**. Good for soft tissue but does not show bone so well.
- **Orbital ultrasound**. Colour Doppler ultrasound to measure size and show bloodflow/velocity within lesion.

KEY POINTS
- Proptosis is axial or non-axial.
- Palpate the orbit to help detect a mass.

28 Orbital and thyroid eye disease

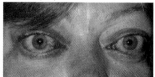

Graves' orbitopathy (thyroid eye disease)

Marked proptosis and redness – active phase

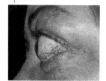

Bilateral proptosis, periorbital swelling and left esotropia – quiet phase

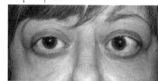

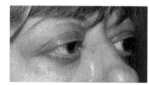

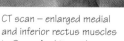

CT scan – enlarged medial and inferior rectus muscles in Graves' orbitopathy

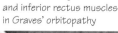

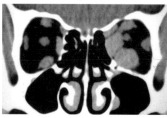

Tumour behind eye

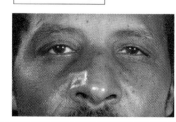

CT scan showing tumour (benign)

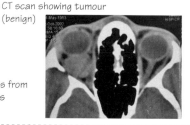

Right proptosis from large cavernous haemangioma

Enucleation Indications for enucleation include a painful blind eye, choroidal malignant melanoma and a severely disrupted eye following trauma.
The eye is eviscerated if there is an intractable endophthalmitis

Post-enucleation socket syndrome – no orbital implant placed at time of enucleation

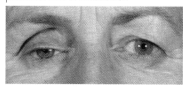

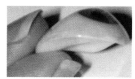

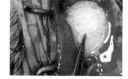

Wearing a thick artificial eye but still very enophthalmic

Thick artificial eye

Porous polyethylene sphere implant inserted into socket.
Orbital sphere implant is needed to replace lost volume

Aims

1 Management of Graves' orbitopathy.
2 Recognize an artificial eye.
This chapter cover proptosis, orbital masses and enucleation.

Common orbital problems

- **Adult**:
  —Graves' orbitopathy (thyroid eye disease) (most common);
  —idiopathic orbital inflammation;
  —cavernous haemangioma;
  —lacrimal gland tumour;
  —secondary tumours;
  —nerve cell or sheath tumours.
- **Child**:
  —dermoid cyst;
  —haemangioma;
  —rhabdomyosarcoma;
  —Craniofacial abnormality.

Graves' orbitopathy

Most patients present within the first 6–12 months of hyperthyroidism. Male patients and smokers have a more aggressive disease. There is an active phase with inflammation which lasts up to 1 year, and a subsequent inactive stable phase. The former is treated medically with immunosuppression (e.g. steroids and azathioprine) and once the disease is inactive surgery to the orbit, muscles and eyelids can be considered.

> **WARNING**
> Early orbital decompression surgery is only done if there is marked compressive optic neuropathy.

There is a varied presentation:
- Proptosis.
- Reduced colour vision from optic nerve compression.
- Restrictive strabismus with mainly inferior and/or medial rectus muscle enlargement causing diplopia.

- Eyelid retraction.
- Lagophthalmos.
- Exposure keratitis.
- Conjunctival redness and cheimosis.
- Periorbital swelling.

The aim of treatment is to preserve vision, with eyes comfortable and looking normal, with full lid closure.

Graves' orbitopathy management

Indication	Phase	Medical treatment	Surgery
Compressive optic neuropathy	Active	• Pulsed steroid therapy • Systemic steroids, azathioprine and orbital radiotherapy	Orbital decompression
Proptosis	Inactive		Orbital decompression
Strabismus	Inactive		Adjustable suture rectus recession
Eyelid retraction	Inactive		• Graduated retractor recession (upper eyelids) • Hard palate mucosal graft, alloderm or auricular cartilage (lower eyelids)
Periorbital swelling	Inactive		Blepharoplasty
Skin changes	Inactive		Laser resurfacing skin

Orbital and lacrimal gland tumours

Orbital and lacrimal gland tumours cause proptosis and require incisional or excisional biopsy by a trained oculoplastics orbital surgeon. Lymphoma and metastases are the commonest malignant tumours.

Many anterior and mid orbital tumours can be biopsied via a skin approach. More posterior intraconal and lacrimal gland tumours (pleomorphic adenoma) require excision via a lateral orbitotomy.

Enucleation

When an eye is removed its volume must be replaced by a buried spherical orbital implant to which the rectus muscles are attached. An ocular prosthesis (artificial eye) is made to match the normal eye; usually it is acrylic and hand painted. If the volume of the enucleated eye is not replaced the patient has a sunken socket appearance called post-enucleation socket syndrome and may need a secondary buried orbital implant.

KEY POINTS

- Graves' orbitopathy—do decompression before eyelid surgery.
- Important to replace eye volume lost at enucleation/evisceration with an orbital implant and artificial eye.

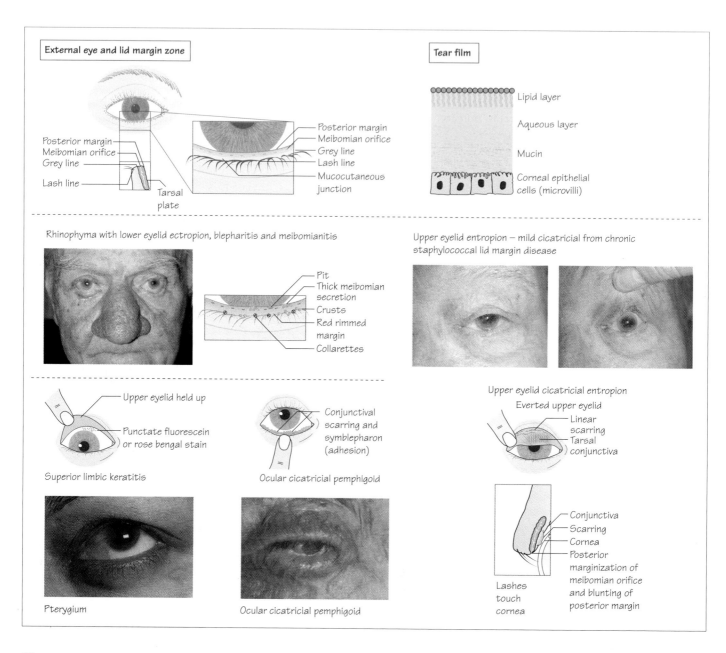

External eye and lid margin zone

Posterior margin
Meibomian orifice
Grey line
Lash line
Tarsal plate

Posterior margin
Meibomian orifice
Grey line
Lash line
Mucocutaneous junction

Tear film

Lipid layer
Aqueous layer
Mucin
Corneal epithelial cells (microvilli)

Rhinophyma with lower eyelid ectropion, blepharitis and meibomianitis

Pit
Thick meibomian secretion
Crusts
Red rimmed margin
Collarettes

Upper eyelid entropion – mild cicatricial from chronic staphylococcal lid margin disease

Upper eyelid cicatricial entropion
Everted upper eyelid

Linear scarring
Tarsal conjunctiva

Upper eyelid held up
Punctate fluorescein or rose bengal stain

Superior limbic keratitis

Conjunctival scarring and symblepharon (adhesion)

Ocular cicatricial pemphigoid

Conjunctiva
Scarring
Cornea
Posterior marginization of meibomian orifice and blunting of posterior margin
Lashes touch cornea

Pterygium

Ocular cicatricial pemphigoid

Aims

Detection and medical management of:
- blepharitis
- dry eyes
- allergic eye disease.

Diseases of the external eye

- Blepharitis.
- Trachoma causing cicatricial entropion.
- Pterygium.
- Allergic eye disease.

Diseases primarily affecting the tear film/epithelium/conjunctiva

- Idiopathic dry eye.
- Severe dry eye associated with Sjögren's syndrome and other autoimmune conditions.
- Graft versus host disease.
- Stevens–Johnson syndrome.
- Ocular cicatricial pemphigoid.

Treatment

Treatment depends on the underlying cause in conjunction with topical lubricating drops. If severe, corneal scarring with superficial vascularization leads to reduced vision and even corneal perforation.

Common conditions

Blepharitis and meibomionitis

Blepharitis

Low-grade chronic staphylococcal lid margin disease with 'red-rimmed' eyelids in young adults and middle-aged persons.

Symptoms

Itchy, sore, watery eyes.

Signs

Red-rimmed lid margins, eyelash crusts and collarettes, and distorted lid margin microanatomy: irregularities, pits and telangiectasia.

Management

• Daily lid hygiene using sodium bicarbonate or dilute baby shampoo and cotton bud lash scrubbing.
• Chloramphenicol ointment, or G fusithalmic
• ±Doxycycline or Minocycline.

Meibomianitis

Thick oily meibomian secretion causing stingy sore eyes and red thickened eyelids. Often associated with rosacea. Management is as for blepharitis, adding tetracycline antibiotic for rosacea.

Upper eyelid entropion

Mild upper eyelid entropion from chronic staphylococcal lid margin disease.

Symptoms

Foreign body lash sensation and dry, gritty eyes.

Signs

Trichiasis and punctate epithelial corneal stain.

Management

• Epilate, electrolysis and cryotherapy trichiasis.
• Topical lubricants.
• Surgery: anterior lamella reposition.

Pterygium (see Chapter 14).

Dry eyes

Idiopathic dry eyes

Symptoms

Gritty, sandy, burning dry eyes with reflex tear flooding (hypersecretion).

Signs

Poor tear film, interpalpebral punctuate epithelial staining, and poor wetting on litmus paper (Schirmer's test).

Management

• Vigorously treat any meibomianitis and blepharitis.
• Artificial tears without preservatives and carbomeric gels.
• Punctal occlusion can be done.

Sjögren's syndrome

Hypofunction of the exocrine glands affecting the lacrimal and salivary glands and the gastrointestinal tract. It affects women in 90% cases, with onset between 35 and 55 years. There is severe fatigue, dry eyes, nose, throat, dental caries and digestive problems. Vision can be impaired from epithelial damage and subsequent conjunctival and corneal scarring. Primary Sjögren's syndrome is idiopathic (approximately 50%) and secondary causes include rheumatoid athritis, lupus or scleroderma.

Other causes of dry eye

• Stevens–Johnson syndrome.
• Ocular cicatricial pemphigoid.
• Lacrimal gland trauma (surgical excision or ductile destruction) and chemical, radiotherapy and thermal injury.
• Fibromyalgia.
• Chronic fatigue syndrome.

Allergic eye disease

• Hayfever: seasonal allergic conjunctivitis. Bilateral, itchy, watery eyes with lid swelling and sometimes mucous discharge. It is a type 1 immediate immune response with histamine release to allergens such as pollen. It is worse in the young with a history of atopy. May also have rhinorrhoea and sneezing. Management is with topical mast cell stabilizer (e.g. sodium chromoglycate or lodoxamide).
• Perennial allergic conjunctivitis. Bilateral, episodic symptoms. Triggered by allergens such as house-dust mites, moulds, pollens, food preservatives and animal danders. Management is as for hayfever, plus oral and topical antihistamine when severe.
• Vernal keratoconjunctivitis sicca (VKC). This is a young person's disease (7–11 years) with characteristic upper tarsal conjunctival cobblestones (see Chapter 23). Also includes bilateral, seasonal, red, puffy, itchy eyes with photophobia, watering and mucous. It may induce ptosis. There are often perilimbal giant papillae, known as limbal vernal. Management is as for hayfever, plus topical steroids when severe.
• Acute allergic conjunctivitis. Sudden, unilateral, itchy lid swelling and marked conjunctival chemosis. Signs are worse than symptoms. Triggered by plant allergens. Resolves spontaneously without treatment within 24–36 h.

Superior limbic keratitis (SLK)

Symptoms

Redness, burning, grittiness, photophobia and frequent blinking.

Signs

Bilateral superior conjunctival punctate stain with fluorescein and rose bengal. The superior limbal conjunctiva is swollen and there may be fine tarsal conjunctival papillae.

Treatment

Treatment is with intense topical lubricant drops.

Ocular cicatricial pemphigoid (OCP)

This severe and fortunately rare conjunctival disease has an insidious onset with redness, grittiness and photophobia (early stages). Later there is cicatricial entropion, severe dry eye, corneal scarring and opacification. There is conjunctival fornix loss with symblepharon and reduction of eye movements. Other mucous membranes may be involved (e.g. mouth, nasal mucosa). Treatment is with systemic immunosuppression, e.g. dapsone.

KEY POINTS

• Blepharitis is a common cause of red-rimmed, itchy eyes.
• Use topical lubricant drops (hypromellose) for dry eyes.
• Excise pterygium only if encroaching onto the cornea and visual axis.

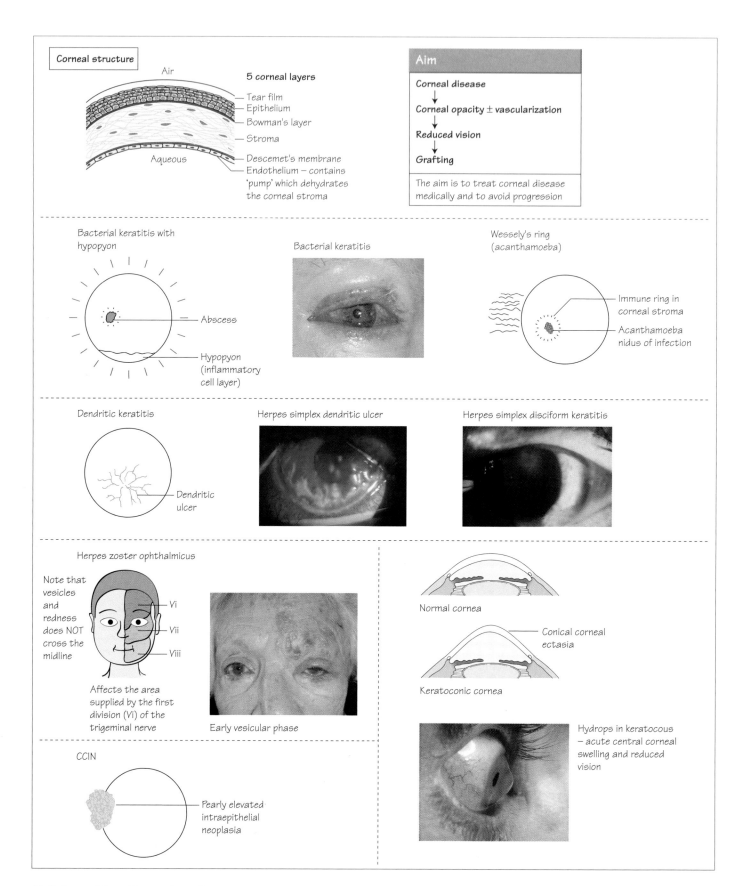

Corneal structure

Air

5 corneal layers
— Tear film
— Epithelium
— Bowman's layer
— Stroma
— Descemet's membrane
— Endothelium — contains 'pump' which dehydrates the corneal stroma

Aqueous

Aim

Corneal disease
↓
Corneal opacity ± vascularization
↓
Reduced vision
↓
Grafting

The aim is to treat corneal disease medically and to avoid progression

Bacterial keratitis with hypopyon

— Abscess

— Hypopyon (inflammatory cell layer)

Bacterial keratitis

Wessely's ring (acanthamoeba)

— Immune ring in corneal stroma
— Acanthamoeba nidus of infection

Dendritic keratitis

— Dendritic ulcer

Herpes simplex dendritic ulcer

Herpes simplex disciform keratitis

Herpes zoster ophthalmicus

Note that vesicles and redness does NOT cross the midline

— Vi
— Vii
— Viii

Affects the area supplied by the first division (Vi) of the trigeminal nerve

Early vesicular phase

Normal cornea

— Conical corneal ectasia

Keratoconic cornea

Hydrops in keratocous — acute central corneal swelling and reduced vision

CCIN

— Pearly elevated intraepithelial neoplasia

Aims

1 Outline the basic anatomy of the cornea.
2 Signs and symptoms of corneal disease.
3 Describe common disease processes involving the cornea.

Corneal clarity

The cornea is a clear because it has a highly organized structure of collagen fibrils, it is free of blood vessels and allows the passage of light in an organized way so a clear image may be focused on the retina. The corneal layers all contribute to its function. The endothelial cells actively pump out fluid from the stroma. A healthy tear film (with all its constituent layers) and eyelids are vital to maintain corneal integrity and clarity.

Disturbance of the eyelids, conjunctiva or tear film may lead to corneal problems including ulceration. If the disease is severe, corneal scarring with vascularization may lead to reduced vision and in rare cases to corneal perforation requiring surgical management. Corneal anaesthesia (Vth nerve palsy) predisposes to severe keratitis.

Corneal disease

Keratitis

General term used to denote inflammation of the cornea from infection and inflammation.

Symptoms
Pain and photosensitivity (maybe absent in herpetic disease due to corneal hypaesthesia), reduced visual acuity and/or discharge.

Signs
Reduced Snellen visual acuity and circumcorneal injection — a red, inflamed eye, presence of staining on fluorescein drop instillation, visible corneal infiltrate with or without anterior chamber hypopyon and blepharospasm.

Infections

Bacterial keratitis
Secondary to minor trauma (corneal abrasion or contact lens wear). *Treat as an emergency.*

A variety of bacteria may be responsible. *Pseudomonas* is common in contact lens-related keratitis and is rapidly destructive. There is rapid corneal opacification and melt over less than 24 h.

Rapidly identify the infective agent by C&S intensive topical antibiotics. Severe infections can lead to corneal perforation, endophthalmitis and loss of vision.

Acanthamoeba keratitis
Acanthamoeba causes prolonged corneal infection. It is associated with poor contact lens hygiene — especially tap water in lens cleaning — and with daily wear soft contact lenses. Characterized by severe pain.

Diagnosis may require corneal biopsy and histological assessment. Look for a corneal Wessely ring using the slit lamp.

Chronic infection with acanthamoeba cysts deep in the corneal stroma may cause scarring requiring corneal graft.

Viral keratitis
1 Herpes simplex types 1 and 2
Epithelial disease — dendritic ulceration.
Stromal disease — disciform keratitis
• immune mediated, presenting as a disc-shaped area of corneal oedema, hence the term disciform;
• stromal necrosis may result in scarring with vascularization reducing corneal sensation, clarity and vision.

Treatment of epithelial disease is with antiviral medication (e.g. aciclovir topically and/or systemically). Judicious use of topical corticosteroids for disciform keratitis.

> **WARNING**
> **Steroid drops.** Do *not* give steroid drops in the presence of active epithelial disease as may cause ulceration and blindness.

2 Herpes zoster ophthalmicus
This affects the Vth cranial nerve with segmental skin vesicles and erythema which includes the upper eyelid. The rash does not cross the forehead midline. There is associated headache, malaise and fever. There is follicular conjunctivitis with variable involvement of the cornea — multiple epithelial pseudodendrites and anterior stromal infiltration — responsive to topical corticosteroids. Increased risk in immunocompromised patients, e.g. HIV. Treatment is with systemic antivirals.

Inflammation

Peripheral necrotizing keratitis
This is related to an underlying systemic vasculitis, e.g. rheumatoid arthritis, systemic lupus erythematosis or Wegener's granulomatosis. Peripheral destruction of corneal tissue is secondary to an ischaemic microvasculitis in the adjacent scleral and conjunctival vessels or it is mediated immunologically by blood-borne factors or matrix metalloproteinases secreted into the tears. This pathological process is exacerbated by secondary Sjögren's syndrome.

Treat the underlying disease process with systemic immunosuppression. Treat corneal perforation conservatively with tissue glue, bandage contact lenses or corneal grafting.

Corneal dystrophies

These are hereditary and occur at any level in the cornea — epithelial, stromal and endothelial. With severe corneal dystrophies, corneal grafting may be required to restore vision, although dystrophic changes often recur in the grafts.

Fingerprint and map-dot corneal epithelial dystrophies cause acute painful recurrent corneal erosions, particularly on waking.

The most common corneal dystrophy, which is potentially sight threatening, is keratoconus — associated with Down's syndrome, disorders of collagen metabolism, atopic eye disease or idiopathic. Keratoconic patients require special fit contact lenses and, if needed, corneal grafting. (See Chapters 31 and 32)

Other dystrophies include lattice dystrophy, with deposition of amyloid in the corneal stroma, and inherited disorders of corneal metabolism (e.g. granular and macular dystrophy).

Fuchs' endothelial dystrophy results in corneal clouding because of endothelial pump failure. It causes a painful bullous keratopathy, which is treated with a bandage contact lens and eventual penetrating keratoplasty.

Corneal neoplasia

Although rare, conjunctival–corneal intraepithelial neoplasia (CCIN) and squamous carcinoma are important conditions. They are more common in fairer-skinned individuals in hotter climes and immunocompromised patients with HIV. Needs to be treated with excision or local destructive procedures.

KEY POINTS
• The healthy cornea is avascular and transparent due to endothelial pump.
• Topical steroids may worsen dendritic keratitis and should never be used.
• Bacterial keratitis in a contact lens wearer is an emergency.

31 Therapeutic contact lenses

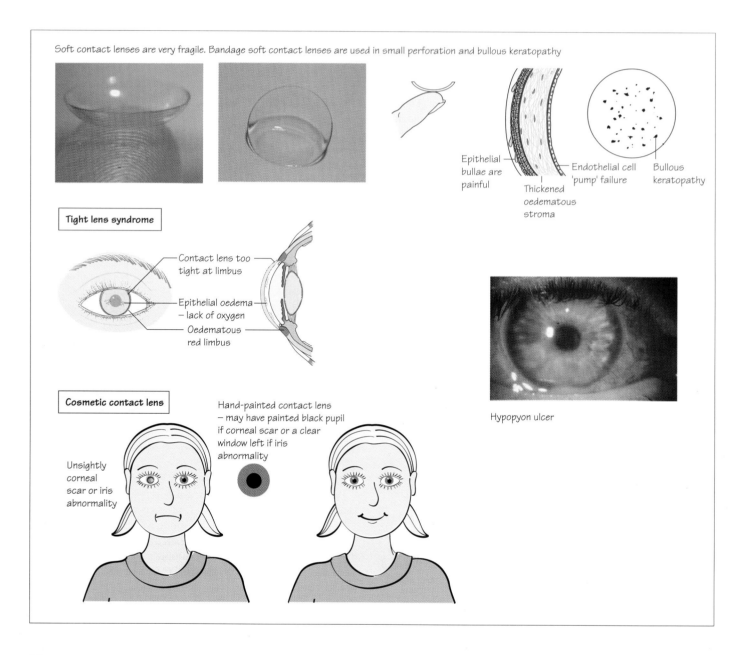

Soft contact lenses are very fragile. Bandage soft contact lenses are used in small perforation and bullous keratopathy

Epithelial bullae are painful

Thickened oedematous stroma

Endothelial cell 'pump' failure

Bullous keratopathy

Tight lens syndrome

Contact lens too tight at limbus

Epithelial oedema – lack of oxygen

Oedematous red limbus

Hypopyon ulcer

Cosmetic contact lens

Hand-painted contact lens – may have painted black pupil if corneal scar or a clear window left if iris abnormality

Unsightly corneal scar or iris abnormality

Aims

1 Medical indications for contact lenses (CL).
2 Complications of contact lens wear.

Contact lenses are an excellent alternative to glasses. They are also widely used therapeutically in corneal disease. They are fitted for each patient based on the steepness and diameter of the cornea. The types of lenses (hard, gas permeable hard, etc.) and materials used are summarized in Chapter 9.

Keratoconus

In keratoconus, (GPH) CL are used. Some soft CL are suitable too in the early stages. Once the corneal curvature is very 'steep' either GPH lenses are used or eventual corneal graft (see Chapter 32).

Therapeutic bandage contact lenses

These are soft contact lenses with several functions.

Protection of normal epithelium

• Trichiasis—to prevent lashes from rubbing the cornea.
• Lid margin deformation, e.g. lower lid entropion with lashes touching the cornea, as temporary relief until surgery can be performed.
• Protection of corneal graft epithelium.
• Dry eye, e.g. pemphigoid and Stevens–Johnson syndrome.
• Exposure keratitis—following seventh nerve palsy.
• To protect the cornea if there are sutures on the lid margin or under the eyelid, abrading the cornea. Use until sutures dissolve or can be removed.

Healing abnormal epithelium

- Corneal epithelial dystrophy, e.g. Cogan's microcystic epithelial dystrophy, Meesman's dystrophy, Reis–Buckler's dystrophy and map-dot or fingerpoint dystrophy.
- Chronic corneal ulcers—due to herpes simplex or vernal keratoconjunctivitis.
- Abrasions and erosions.
- Filamentary keratitis—also rapid relief of the discomfort caused by the corneal filaments.
- Chemical, thermal and irradiation burns—high water content lenses may be useful to restore normal epithelialization.

Moulding and splinting

- Post keratoplasty (corneal grafting)—to flatten and reposition the graft when lifting or displacement of graft occurs.
- Wound leaks—small corneal perforations need tight fitting; post-trabeculectomy bleb leaks need large lenses to cover the leak.

Pain relief

- Bullous keratopathy—CL help to alleviate pain by covering exposed nerve endings.
- Postrefractive surgery—PRK and LASEK for pain relief and wound healing. See Chapter 32.

Complications of contact lenses
Corneal physiology

The constant metabolic activity in the cornea maintains transparency, temperature, cell reproduction and the transport of tissue materials. The main nutrients are glucose, amino acids (from the aqueous humour) and oxygen (from the tear film by diffusion when the eye is open and from the tarsal conjunctiva when the eyelids are closed). Without oxygen there is hypoxia or anoxia.

Hypoxia and anoxia
There are virtually no lenses available that fully meet the oxygen requirements of the cornea, and there is no CL as physiological or oxygen permeable as having no CL on the eye!

One of the first important effects of **hypoxia** (which the patient is unaware of) is a drop in corneal sensitivity. **Anoxia** causes corneal swelling, especially of the epithelium. If there is not enough oxygen available to convert glucose, by the means of glycolysis, into energy, the waste product (lactic acid) is allowed to diffuse and build up in the stroma. Sufficient osmotic pressure is created to allow water to be drawn into the stroma faster than the endothelial pump can remove it, so eventually corneal epithelial and stromal swelling occurs.

Lack of oxygen results in:
- Acute epithelial necrosis.
- Microcystic epitheliopathy.
- Epithelial and stromal oedema.
- Corneal neovascularization.

Anatomical effects

Anatomical effects result in:
- Tight lens syndrome.
- Corneal abrasions (foreign bodies).

- Three and 9 o'clock staining (drying of corneal surface, abnormal blink).
- Inferior corneal stain (incomplete blinking).
- Dimple veil (static air bubble under lens).
- Overwearing syndrome (mechanical and metabolic factors).

Biological activity

The presence of a CL acting as a biological active surface can cause several syndromes:
- Toxic keratopathy (proteolytic enzyme—the chemical preservative in the cleaning solutions).
- Thiomersal keratopathy (the preservative in CL solutions or instilled eye drops acts as a hapten causing a delayed hypersensitivity response).
- Giant papillary conjunctivitis (multifactorial aetiology—immune response to antigenic proteins on lenses and mechanical effects of lens edge) causes red sticky eye.
- Sterile corneal infiltrate—inflammatory response in absence of infecting organism, hypersensitivity to disinfectants and bacterial products as well as lens fit are aetiological factors.

Microbial keratitis

This is caused by a complex interaction of various factors and increased ocular susceptibility and exposure to pathogens, associated with *Pseudomonas*, *Staphylococcus* and *Acanthamoeba* (ubiquitous free-living protozon).

Guidelines for managing microbial conjunctivitis
Emergencies are a routine occurrence in CL practice.

> **WARNING**
> In a contact lens wearer corneal and conjunctival complications are due to contact lens wear until proved otherwise.

- *Leave the lens out*—Inflammatory symptoms of lens-related disease respond within a few days of ceasing lens wear.
- *Exclude microbial keratitis.*
- *Do not treat a red eye with steroids when there is a corneal ulcer.*

Advice for patients

Maintain a high standard of CL hygiene. Lenses should be cleaned and disinfected each time they are removed. Avoid overnight wear! Have back up spectacles! Leave lenses out when adverse symptoms or a red eye develops.

> *Feel good—look good—see good*, if these critieria are not met the patient should seek help.

KEY POINTS
- Use bandage CL for corneal protection, to aid healing, splinting and pain relief.
- Anoxia causes corneal swelling, cloudiness and pain.
- Beware bacterial contact lens complications!

32 Corneal and laser photorefractive surgery

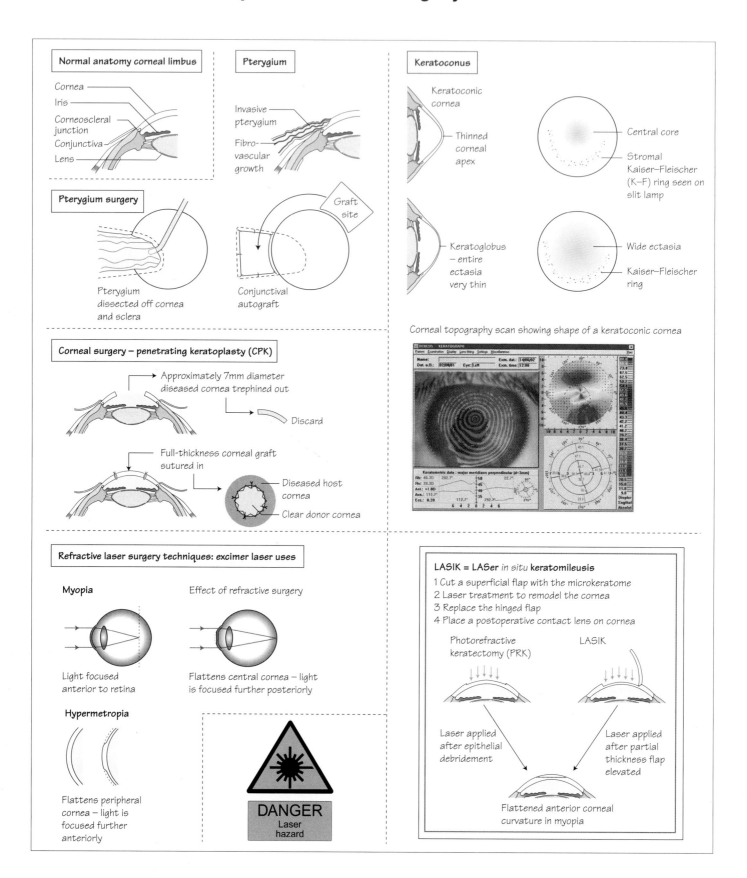

Normal anatomy corneal limbus

Cornea
Iris
Corneoscleral junction
Conjunctiva
Lens

Pterygium

Invasive pterygium
Fibro-vascular growth

Pterygium surgery

Graft site

Pterygium dissected off cornea and sclera

Conjunctival autograft

Keratoconus

Keratoconic cornea

Thinned corneal apex

Keratoglobus – entire ectasia very thin

Central core

Stromal Kaiser–Fleischer (K–F) ring seen on slit lamp

Wide ectasia

Kaiser–Fleischer ring

Corneal topography scan showing shape of a keratoconic cornea

Corneal surgery – penetrating keratoplasty (CPK)

Approximately 7mm diameter diseased cornea trephined out

Discard

Full-thickness corneal graft sutured in

Diseased host cornea

Clear donor cornea

Refractive laser surgery techniques: excimer laser uses

Myopia

Effect of refractive surgery

Light focused anterior to retina

Flattens central cornea – light is focused further posteriorly

Hypermetropia

Flattens peripheral cornea – light is focused further anteriorly

DANGER
Laser hazard

LASIK = LASer in situ keratomileusis

1 Cut a superficial flap with the microkeratome
2 Laser treatment to remodel the cornea
3 Replace the hinged flap
4 Place a postoperative contact lens on cornea

Photorefractive keratectomy (PRK)

LASIK

Laser applied after epithelial debridement

Laser applied after partial thickness flap elevated

Flattened anterior corneal curvature in myopia

Aims

1 Management of keratoconus.
2 Principles of corneal surgery.
3 Know about current laser techniques.

Cornea

The healthy cornea is clear, tough and free of blood vessels or opacification and acts as an important refractive surface. Corneal clarity is dependent on the integrity and normal functioning of all of its 5 cellular layers (see Chapter 30). Of particular importance is the corneal endothelium, a single cell layer of non-mitotic cells that maintains the cornea in a state of partial 'dehydration' and hence transparency through the use of cellular metabolic 'pumps'. When that pump fails, the stroma swells and becomes hazy, e.g. bullous keratopathy (see Chapter 31) requiring bandage CL or full thickness corneal graft (penetrating keratoplasty, PK).

Keratitis causing corneal scarring can require PK. In order for the graft to take, the host cornea should not have many blood vessels, which could contribute to corneal graft rejection, and should have near or near normal sensation. A partial thickness corneal graft is a lamellar keratoplasty.

Corneal diseases

Keratoconus

This common corneal dystrophy is a chronic progressive disease characterized by thinning, cone formation and irregular myopic astigmatism (see Chapter 30). The criteria for diagnosis are steep keratometric readings with irregular light reflexes on the corneal surface seen with the keratoscope and corneal topography.

Early management is with SPH CL, and late management with PK.

Pterygium

Microscopic lamella excision is needed if it encroaches on the visual axis (See Chapter 14.)

Corneal neoplasia (See Chapter 30)

Corneal surgery

Corneal grafting

From human donor material. Donor eyes are stored in eye banks e.g. in London, Bristol, Manchester and Dublin. Donors are screened for many contagious diseases including HIV.

Indications
• Visual rehabilitation following scarring, dystrophic changes or endothelial dysfunction resulting in loss of corneal clarity.
• Restoration of structural integrity following perforation.
• Alleviation of pain in intractable corneal disease without visual potential, e.g. bullous keratopathy.

Refractive surgery

Surgery and/or laser is used to reshape the main refractive surface of the eye, (anterior corneal surface), and to bring light rays in focus on the retina without the need for glasses or contact lenses.

The main indication is **myopia**.

There are three methods of laser, in all of which the **excimer laser** is used to correct myopia, hypermetropia and astigmatism under local anaesthesia.

In myopia the corneal surface is flattened so that the image focuses onto the retina. The effect in hypermetropia is not always stable.

Photorefractive keratectomy (PRK)

Excimer laser ablation reshapes the anterior corneal surface after manual debridement of the epithelium. >10 years' track record.
• Suitable for low refractive errors (−1 to −6D).
• Disappointing for hypermetropia.
• Bandage contact lenses as eye painful for 48h.
• Variable slow healing and remodelling over months.
• Quality of vision—temporary haze common after treatment.
• Regression can occur in higher degrees of myopia (>−10D).
• Recurrent erosions are a complication.

Laser-assisted in intrastromal in situ keratomileusis (LASIK)

A partial thickness corneal hinged epithelial 'cap' is raised and the excimer laser ablation is applied to stromal tissue below this, after which the 'cap' is replaced. <10 years' track record.
• Suitable for higher degrees of myopia with less risk of regression (up to −10D).
• Disappointing for hypermetropia.
• No haze.
• Best visual acuity achieved more rapidly than PRK.
• Dry eye for a few months.

Laser epithelium keratomileusis (LASEK)

This is large optical zone corneal surface excimer laser ablation. The epithelium is treated with 15% alcohol for 20s and is preserved or delaminated with a microkeratome and is later replaced. This is the newest technique with a short track record, 5 yrs.
• A bandage contact lens is worn for 3–4 days whilst the epithelium heals.
• There is speedy healing because the epithelium is retained.
• Mild pain only.
• Good for astigmatism.
• Excellent for myopia ≤6D, good for myopia −6 to ≤10D, allright for myopia −10 to −12D and for hypermetropia up to +4D.
• Studies have limited follow-up data, often <2 years.
• Less haze risk than in PRK.

Who can have laser refractive surgery?

• Patients should be >21 years, have a stable refraction, not pregnant and have no keratoconus, cataract or glaucoma.
• They should not be on systemic steroids.
• Patients should have realistic expectations and have been warned of potential side effects of haze, night time glare, ghosting images, starburst around lights, dry eye and risk of macular haemorrhage.
• It is also essential that patients are warned that intraocular pressure and A-scan/biometry measurements cannot be made accurately after refractive surgery.

WARNING

1 Corneal refractive surgery can have serious, potentially sight-threatening complications as with any ocular surgery.
2 Lasered donor eyes are not accepted for corneal grafting.
3 Refractive surgery effects may regress with time.

KEY POINTS

• A healthy corneal endothelium is essential for corneal clarity.
• Corneal grafting is successful particularly in keratoconus patients.
• The main indication for laser refractive surgery is myopia.

33 Cataract assessment

Anatomy

The **lens** is crystalline with an inner nucleus of older inactive cells and an outer cortex, the whole being encapsulated. The **epithelium** is active metabolically, it synthesizes protein for **lens fibres**, transports amino acids and maintains a cation pump to keep the lens clear. At the equator of the lens, epithelial cells differentiate into lens fibres, which lose their organelles and ability for aerobic metabolism

Zonule filaments suspend the lens **ciliary processes** to the **ciliary muscle**. When the muscle contracts the filaments relax allowing the lens to become more convex with a shorter focal length for reading

Definition

Cataract: Opacity of the lens of the eye, which occurs when fluid gathers between the lens fibres. The refractive index alters and causes light scatter with resultant blurred vision. Acquired lens changes occur in 95% of people over 65, however, not all these people will require cataract surgery

Diagram of normal anterior segment

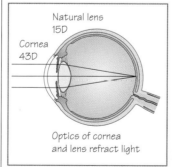

Close up of normal lens cross-section

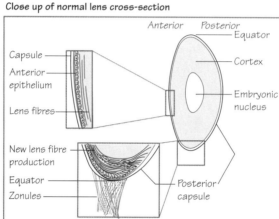
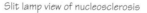

Lens with cataract

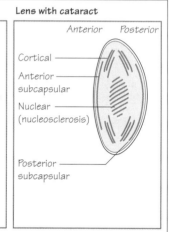

Causes of cataract

- Old age (commonest)
- Associated with other ocular and systemic diseases (diabetes, uveitis, previous ocular surgery)
- Associated with systemic medication (steroids, phenothiazines)
- Trauma and intraocular foreign bodies
- Ionizing radiation (X-ray, UV)
- Congenital (dominant, sporadic or part of a syndrome, abnormal galactose metabolism, hypoglycaemia)
- Associated with inherited abnormality (myotonic dystrophy, Marfan's syndrome, Lowe's syndrome, rubella, high myopia)

Slit lamp view of nucleosclerosis

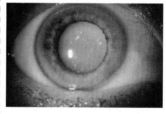
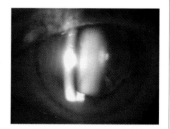

Biometry: intraocular lens power calculation

The desired implant should produce a sharp image on the retina. Since each eye has a different corneal curvature and axial length, the implant size has to be measured preoperatively in each patient. The optics of the eye are such that light is refracted by the cornea (effective power of 43D) and by the natural lens (effective power 15D), both of these together give the total power of the focusing components of the eye. A special equation is used to calculate the intraocular lens power, which is usually in the range of 19–22D, with some very short-sighted eyes needing lower powers and long-sighted eyes needing higher powers for clear focused distance vision

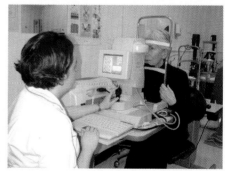

Natural lens 15D
Cornea 43D
Optics of cornea and lens refract light

Aims

1 Anatomy of the lens.
2 Causes of cataract.
3 Symptoms and signs.
4 Treatment of cataract.

Cataract is the most common cause of blindness in adults worldwide.

Symptoms

- Reduced visual acuity (near and distant objects).
- Glare in sunshine or with street or car lights.
- Distortion of lines.
- Monocular diplopia.
- Altered colours (white objects appear yellowish).
- Not associated with pain, discharge or redness of the eye.

Signs

- Reduced acuity measured on a Snellen chart or LogMar and near vision chart.
- An abnormally dim red reflex is seen when the retina is viewed with an ophthalmoscope at arms length. Nuclear cataract causes a central black shadow across the red reflex and cortical cataracts cause black spoke-like shadows coming from the edge of the red reflex.
- Reduced contrast sensitivity can be measured by the ophthalmologist.
- Only very dense cataracts causing severely impaired vision cause a white pupil.
- After pupils have been dilated, slit lamp examination shows whether the cataract is cortical, nuclear or posterior subcapsular and allows fundus examination.
- Cataract in children is unusual but may be associated with a white pupil, inability to fix on a target (e.g. a light) and the development of a squint.

TIP
Pupils are normal if there is no other ocular or optic nerve disease.

Treatment

- Cataract alters the refractive power of the natural lens so a change in glasses prescription may allow good vision to be maintained. The eye may become more myopic (lenticular-induced myopia) or hyperopic. The legal requirement for driving a car in the UK is 6/10 in one eye. NB, the Snellen chart only has lines corresponding to 6/9 and 6/12.
- If further changes occur in the lens, with increased disturbance of the lens fibres, the visual acuity cannot be improved with glasses and surgical removal of the cataractous lens is required.
- Modern surgery involves removal of the lens fibres, which form the nucleus and cortex of the cataract, leaving the posterior epithelial capsule to hold the new artificial lens and keep the vitreous humour away from the anterior chamber.

Preparation for cataract surgery

- Biometry: ultrasound measurement of the length of the eye and keratometry to measure the curvature of the cornea and hence calculate the power of the implant to be inserted in the eye during surgery.
- Confirm that general health problems are stable, particularly hypertension, respiratory disease and diabetes.
- Some medication increases the incidence of haemorrhage. Warfarin does not need to be stopped but the INR should be less than 3. Aspirin may be stopped 1 week before surgery.
- Inform patients of expected outcome and the complications of surgery (informed consent).

KEY POINTS

- Cataract is common, it is one of the three main causes of blindness worldwide.
- Can occur at any age and in all races.
- Effectively treated by glasses in the early stages and by surgery when more advanced.

34 Cataract surgery

An operating microscope is needed. In order to reach the lens, a small corneal incision is made close to the limbus for the phaco-probe. It is important to appreciate ANTERIOR CHAMBER DEPTH and to keep all instruments away from the corneal endothelium, in the plane of the iris

Model of eye showing anterior chamber depth

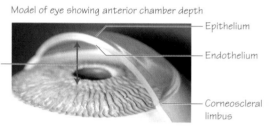

- Epithelium
- Endothelium
- Corneoscleral limbus

Anterior chamber depth

Phacoemulsification surgery

1. Keratome corneal incision

3. Foldable intraocular lens (IOL) being inserted

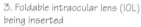

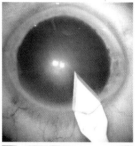
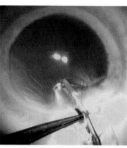

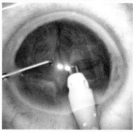

2. Phaco-probe sculpting lens nucleus

4. IOL unfolded in capsular bag

Phaco-probe

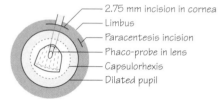

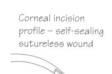

- 2.75 mm incision in cornea
- Limbus
- Paracentesis incision
- Phaco-probe in lens
- Capsulorhexis
- Dilated pupil

Corneal incision profile – self-sealing sutureless wound

Intraocular lens

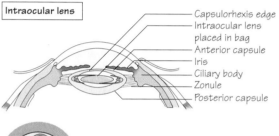

- Capsulorhexis edge
- Intraocular lens placed in bag
- Anterior capsule
- Iris
- Ciliary body
- Zonule
- Posterior capsule

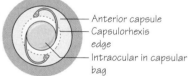

- Anterior capsule
- Capsulorhexis edge
- Intraocular in capsular bag

Steps:
- Corneal incision 2.75–3.2 mm
- Viscoelastic to anterior chamber
- Capsulorhexis
- Hydrodissection
- Phaco removal of nucleus
- Aspiration of cortex
- More viscoelastic:
- A folded IOL is inserted under a cushion of viscoelastic fluid, which protects the corneal endothelium; the lens unfolds spontaneously within the capsular bag
- Viscoelastic removed and replaced with balanced salt solution
- Self-sealing wound
- Subconjunctival injection of steroid and antibiotic
- Eyepad and protective eye shield

New techniques
Clear lens surgery – a novel lens refractive technique

Phacoemulsification is used for cataract surgery and also for CLEAR LENS surgery. Clear lens surgery is called lens refractive surgery and is increasingly being offered for presbyopia and high myopia. Technology for lens surgery is accelerating at a phenomenal speed

1. Clear lens IOL – the patient's lens is removed and an IOL of a different power inserted. E.g. Prelex lens exchange – this is a special IOL which tilts with accommodation maintaining clear 'unaided' distance and near vision! Myopic patients having LASER corneal refractive surgery now may opt for this when prebyopic!

2. Phakic IOL – the patient's clear lens is left *in situ* and a second lens placed in front of it – used for myopia correction

Both these techniques have potential complications and the patient needs to be fully informed before going ahead

Aims

1 Understand methods of anaesthesia and cataract removal.
2 Be able to explain cataract surgery to a patient.

Microsurgical cataract surgery in developed countries has reached a very high level due to the developments in microsurgical instruments and intraocular lens design. There is controlled and precise removal of part of the lens with the assistance of an operating microscope. Part of the lens capsule is retained to hold the implant within it.

Definitions

Pseudophakia: An eye that has had a cataract removed and artificial intraocular lens implanted.
Aphakia: An eye that has had a cataract removed without an artificial lens inserted.

Anaesthesia for cataract surgery

> **TIP**
> Most adult cataract surgery is done under topical or local anaesthesia. The patient may see bright lights and different colours, shadows of the surgeon's hands moving or complete darkness during surgery.

Local anaesthesia

- Topical (drops of proxymethocaine or amethocaine).
- Subtenons using a blunt canula to administer 2 ml of lidocaine.
- Peribulbar injection to distribute 5–10 ml lidocaine within the orbit.
- Retrobulbar injection to direct 1–2 ml lidocaine within the muscle cone—now becoming less commonly used.

Sedation

Intravenous drugs may be given with local anaesthetics but are not preferred as the patient could drift off to sleep and then suddenly wake up with a jolt and move their head—undesirable in cataract surgery.

General anaesthesia

This is used for young and uncooperative patients.

Surgical technique for cataract removal

Patients have to lie supine so a microscope with a bright light and good magnification can be positioned above them. The surgeon works from the side or above the head, looking down the microscope, using the red reflex from the retina to aid cataract removal.

Draping

Before surgery can start, the eyelids and lashes are covered with a thin transparent plastic drape in order to keep contaminated lashes out of the surgical field. Staphylococci live in abundance on the lashes. The drape is light and also covers the face—lifted up from it as a small tent—to protect the face from irrigation fluids used in the surgery, which are collected into a small bag at the side of the head.

Small speculum

The eyelids are kept open by a combination of the drape and a small wire speculum which does not cause the patient discomfort.

> **TIP**
> Phacoemulsification lens surgery with small, foldable intraocular lens implants is the gold standard. It gives rapid visual rehabilitation with a low complication rate.

Surgery

Extracapsular cataract surgery is a technique in which the posterior capsule of the lens is retained, keeping the vitreous separate from the anterior chamber of the eye. It may be small or large incision surgery.

- **Small incision surgery** is by using phacoemulsification (phaco) to crumble the lens in the eye. Fragments are irrigated out automatically. A soft, foldable intraocular lens implant (IOL) can be inserted through the small incision into the lens capsule (posterior chamber IOL). This incision is usually sutureless, or a single suture is placed, which can be removed as early as 2 weeks after surgery. Phaco is the most commonly used technique.
- **Large incision surgery** involves removal of the entire nucleus as one piece; the soft cortex is aspirated and a rigid or soft implant is inserted. The corneal wound requires microsutures, which are removed as late as 8 weeks after surgery.

Implant power

The IOL power is carefully calculated to take into account the patients postoperative visual requirements. For instance, a myopic person may prefer to remain slightly myopic after surgery so that they can still read without glasses. Multifocal IOLs and accommodative IOLs are increasingly being used.

Clear lens surgery for presbyopia

Over the next few years an increasing number of people in their fifties will have their lenses removed for presbyopia, in order to avoid having to wear reading glasses, and special accommodative IOLs will be inserted. Hence the number of people developing cataract will be reduced.

KEY POINTS

- Microsurgery involving the replacment of the natural lens with an artificial one.
- Day-case procedure under local anaesthesia.
- Patient needs to be able to lie still and flat for 30 min.

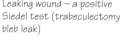

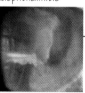

Leaking wound – a positive Siedel test (trabeculectomy bleb leak)

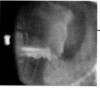

Hypopyon indicates endophthalmitis

Fibrin plaque – intense postoperative inflammation in endophthalitis

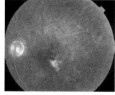

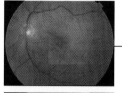

Cystoid macular oedema (CMO) – typical colour fundus and fluorescein angiographic appearance

Early postoperative problems	Symptom	Sign	Treatment
Raised intraocular pressure	Pain, deep ache, blurred vision	Hazy cornea	Ophthalmologist needs to measure pressure and treat with systemic acetazolamide 250 mg 2–4 times daily (1–2 days) and glaucoma drops
Leaking incision	Poor vision	Siedel positive with fluorescein	Ophthalmologist may need to suture the wound in the operating theatre. If the anterior chamber is deep and the ocular pressure is normal, a soft contact lens may be placed on the eye. Daily review is required
Subconjunctival haemorrhage	Red eye. No pain	Diffuse redness on the globe	Continue drops. Reinforce good technique for instilling drops
Corneal oedema	Poor vision	Hazy cornea	Ophthalmologist needs to exclude raised pressure and increase topical steroid drops
Epithelial erosion (conjunctiva or cornea)	Gritty, watering	Fluorescein staining, may have injected bulbar conjunctiva	Continue drops, reassure. Monitor carefully to exclude early infection
Conjunctivitis	Pain, redness with mucopurulent discharge	Swollen, red tarsal conjunctiva while maintaining good vision	Prescribe different antibiotic, (e.g. ofloxacin) to be used 2 hourly. Frequent review to confirm no progression to endophthalmitis

Sight-threatening postop problems requiring urgent treatment by ophthalmologist	Symptom	Signs observed with pen torch	Slit lamp signs observed by ophthalmologist	Treatment (by ophthalmologist)
Endophthalmitis	Painful, red eye usually with a mucopurulent discharge and poor vision at day 3–5	Red eye with hazy cornea. A relative afferent pupillary defect indicates serious visual damage	Flare, cells and and hypopyon in anterior chamber	URGENT in-patient management. Intensive topical broad spectrum antibiotics (drops). Requires aqueous and vitreous sample for microscopy, culture and sensitivity
Macular oedema (retina)	Poor vision during first 60 days after surgery	Normal anterior segment of the eye	Slit lamp fundus examination and fluorescein angiography show increased fluid in the retina around the fovea	Treated with anti-inflammatory drops (steroid and non-steroidal), steroid injection around the eye, systemic non-steroidal anti-inflammatory, e.g. neurofen
Opacity of posterior part of the original epithelial capsule of the natural lens (can occur between 1 month and 2 years after surgery)	Gradual deterioration of vision, as though cataract is reforming	White eye with no external abnormality. Red reflex from fundus may be obscured	Posterior capsule hazy or white. Implant is unaffected	Make a hole in the capsule using a YAG laser (clinic procedure requiring anaesthetic drops). Cornea, anterior chamber and implant are not affected by the laser

Definitions:
Endophthalmitis = infection and inflammation involving the whole of the contents of the eyeball
IOP = Intraocular pressure
YAG laser capsulotomy = laser treatment for posterior capsular opacity
Siedel test = fluorescein test to look for wound leakage of aqueous humour from the eye

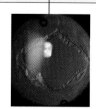

YAG capsulotomy hole made in thickened posterior capsule

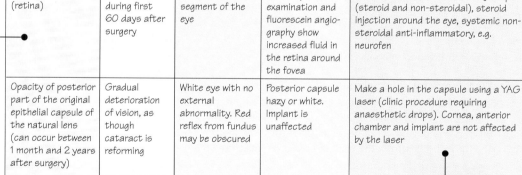

Aims

1 Awareness of normal and undesirable early and late postoperative events.

2 Recognize postop complications from history.

3 Use of pen torch and fluorescein drops to detect a leaking wound and see hypopyon.

Routine postoperative management

Patients use steroid and antibiotic drops four times daily for 2–4 weeks after surgery. During that time they can read, take gentle exercise, shop, shower or bath and wash their hair carefully. The implant inserted at surgery normally gives them clear vision for distance (e.g. TV, buses) but they will need to wear reading glasses (approximate prescription +2.5D); these can be prescribed from 2–4 weeks after phacocataract surgery. Some patients have a multifocal implant inserted so they are less dependent on glasses for reading.

Reading glasses

Patients who have had phacocataract surgery usually have good vision from the first postoperative day and can be tested for spectacles (refraction) for reading 2 weeks after surgery.

In contrast, patients who have had large excision extracapsular cataract surgery have corneal sutures, which are not removed for 2–3 months. Only after these have been removed are reading spectacles prescribed, i.e. there is a longer rehabilitation period.

Undesirable postoperative events (complications)

Watering and a foreign body sensation are common after surgery. Usually the patient can be reassured, but the possibility of infection—**endophthalmitis**—the most important sight-threatening complication, must be considered. This is an acute sight-threatening postoperative event that requires *urgent* admission and treatment. Its onset is usually 4–5 days after surgery. Symptoms include worsening vision and pain.

See Tables for early and late complications.

KEY POINTS

- Over 97% of cataract surgery is successful.
- Endophthalmitis is the most serious postoperative complication.
- Sympathetic ophthalmia affects the other eye—*rare* <0.01%.

36 Glaucoma—the basics

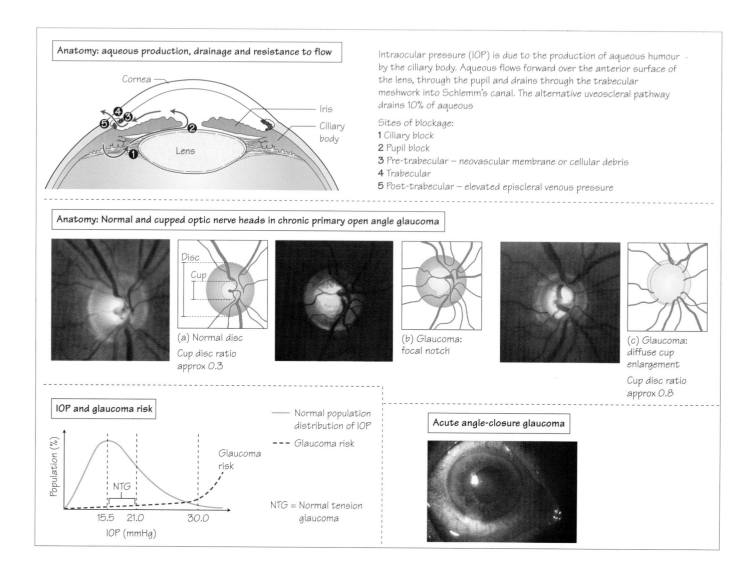

Anatomy: aqueous production, drainage and resistance to flow

Cornea

Iris

Ciliary body

Lens

Intraocular pressure (IOP) is due to the production of aqueous humour by the ciliary body. Aqueous flows forward over the anterior surface of the lens, through the pupil and drains through the trabecular meshwork into Schlemm's canal. The alternative uveoscleral pathway drains 10% of aqueous

Sites of blockage:
1 Ciliary block
2 Pupil block
3 Pre-trabecular – neovascular membrane or cellular debris
4 Trabecular
5 Post-trabecular – elevated episcleral venous pressure

Anatomy: Normal and cupped optic nerve heads in chronic primary open angle glaucoma

Disc

Cup

(a) Normal disc

Cup disc ratio approx 0.3

(b) Glaucoma: focal notch

(c) Glaucoma: diffuse cup enlargement

Cup disc ratio approx 0.8

IOP and glaucoma risk

Population (%)

—— Normal population distribution of IOP

- - - Glaucoma risk

Glaucoma risk

NTG

15.5 21.0 30.0

IOP (mmHg)

NTG = Normal tension glaucoma

Acute angle-closure glaucoma

Aims
1 Understand the group of conditions classed as glaucoma.
2 Know the symptoms and signs of acute angle-closure glaucoma to enable urgent referral for treatment of this ophthalmic emergency.

Definitions
Glaucoma: A multifactorial optic neuropathy with characteristic acquired loss of optic nerve fibres. Commonest cause of irreversible blindness in the world, affecting 2% of people over 40 years of age, and 4% of people over 70 years.
Intraocular pressure (IOP): The 'normal' range of IOP varies between 10 and 21 mmHg but there is no absolute limit. Elevated IOP is a major risk factor for the development of glaucoma.

Skills to obtain
Use of direct ophthalmoscope to evaluate optic disc colour and cup : disc ratio.

Classification
The glaucomas are a diverse group of eye conditions (at least 60 types), which can be divided into diagnostic groups in the following way:
1 Defined by absence or presence of causative factors: **primary** or **secondary**.
2 Defined by the anatomy of the drainage angle: **open angle** or **angle closure**.
3 Defined by speed of onset: **acute** or **chronic**.
4 Defined by age of onset: **congenital**, **juvenile** or **adult**.
5 Defined by level of IOP: **normal tension glaucoma** (characteristic glaucomatous optic neuropathy with IOP in the normal range) or **ocular hypertension** (IOP above the normal range but no glaucomatous optic neuropathy).

Chronic primary open-angle glaucoma (POAG)
This is by far the commonest form of glaucoma in Caucasian and Afro-Caribbean populations. The exact mechanism of pathogene-

sis is unknown, but various factors are implicated including elevated IOP and altered vascular supply to the optic nerve. Genetics also plays a role, with nine loci in the human genome known to be associated with glaucoma. Risk factors include elevated IOP, family history and Afro-Caribbean descent.

Symptoms
Usually asymptomatic until disease is advanced with advanced optic disc cupping, when peripheral field defect may be noticed and central vision lost. 'Tunnel' vision is not noticed early on.

Signs
- Usually raised IOP >21 and <40 mmHg.
- Normal open angle on gonioscopy.
- Characteristic optic disc changes with gradual thinning of the neurosensory rim superiorly and inferiorly with time, nerve fibre layer defect, optic disc rim notching and cupping, cup:disc ratio enlarged and/or asymmetrical.
- Visual field changes on automated fields analysis with characteristic arcuate scotoma.

Treatment
- Medical with daily or twice daily topical drops, laser and surgical options (see Chapter 38 for details).
- Most patients are maintained on regular topical medication with monitoring of disc appearance and visual field analysis.

Acute angle-closure glaucoma (AACG)
Commoner in older, hypermetropic people. Commonest glaucoma in Chinese people.

Symptoms
- Sudden onset of severly painful red eye.
- Blurred vision.
- Halos around lights.
- Headache.
- ±Nausea and vomiting.

> **WARNING**
> Patients with AACG can go blind if the glaucoma is unrecognized and untreated.

Signs
- Reduced visual acuity.
- Brick red eye.
- Hazy cornea (corneal oedema).
- Vertically mid-dilated fixed pupil.
- Very high IOP, that can be felt digitally.
- Closed iridocorneal angle on gonioscopy.

Treatment
Urgent treatment needed to prevent permanent loss of vision.
- Treat medically (topical and systemic) to bring down IOP and break attack.
- Prevent further attacks with YAG laser iridotomy or surgical peripheral iridectomy (in both eyes).
- The second eye is treated prophylactically to prevent later AACG (see Chapter 38).

Secondary glaucoma
Multiple causes including uveitis, rubeofis and trauma.

Treatment
Treat the cause and control IOP.

Chronic angle-closure glaucoma
Younger age group with intermittent angle-closure symptoms.

Treatment
Laser peripheral iridotomy.

Congenital glaucoma / infantile glaucoma / buphthalmos
Occurs in infancy, and can be unilateral or bilateral. Primary or associated with ocular malformation or systemic syndrome, e.g. Sturge–Weber. Can go blind if not detected and treated.

Symptoms
Watering photophobic eyes.

Signs
- Large eyes (myopic)—buphthalmos.
- Diameter of corneas wider than normal.
- Reduced vision.
- Clouding of corneas.
- Linear tears in Descemet's membrane.
- Raised IOP.
- ± Red eyes.

Treatment
- Specialist medical management by paediatric ophthalmologist.
- Then various surgeries, goniotomy, trabeculotomy or trabeculectomy.
- Goniotomy is the first choice and may have to be repeated.

KEY POINTS
- Normal range of intraocular pressure is 10–21 mmHg.
- Primary open-angle glaucoma is the commonest form.
- Acute angle-closure glaucoma occurs in older persons and is usually painful.

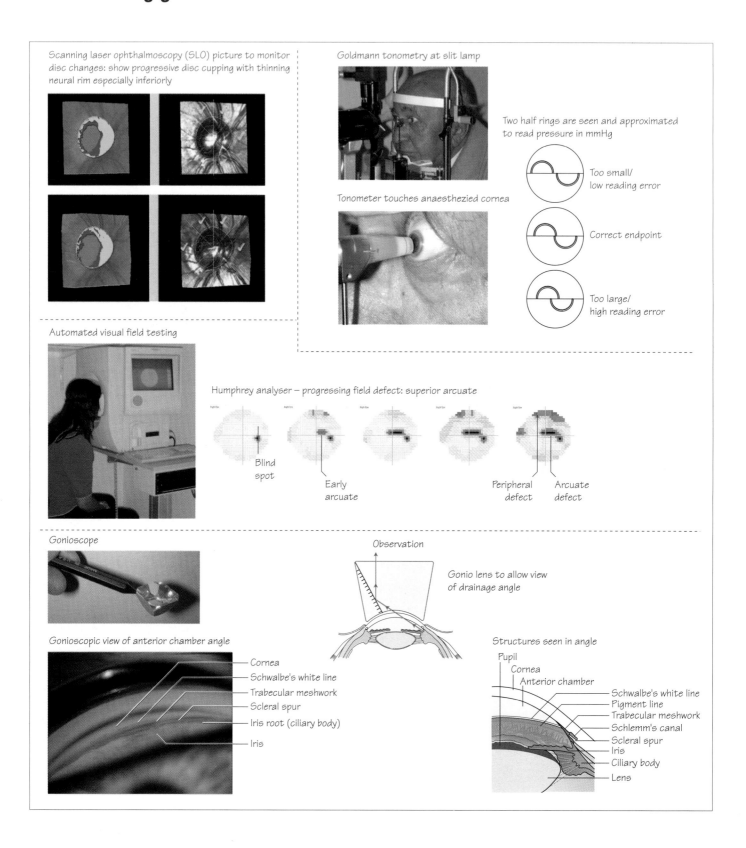

Scanning laser ophthalmoscopy (SLO) picture to monitor disc changes: show progressive disc cupping with thinning neural rim especially inferiorly

Goldmann tonometry at slit lamp

Two half rings are seen and approximated to read pressure in mmHg

Too small/ low reading error

Correct endpoint

Too large/ high reading error

Tonometer touches anaesthezied cornea

Automated visual field testing

Humphrey analyser – progressing field defect: superior arcuate

Blind spot

Early arcuate

Peripheral defect

Arcuate defect

Gonioscope

Observation

Gonio lens to allow view of drainage angle

Gonioscopic view of anterior chamber angle

— Cornea
— Schwalbe's white line
— Trabecular meshwork
— Scleral spur
— Iris root (ciliary body)
— Iris

Structures seen in angle

Pupil
Cornea
Anterior chamber

— Schwalbe's white line
— Pigment line
— Trabecular meshwork
— Schlemm's canal
— Scleral spur
— Iris
— Ciliary body
— Lens

Aim

Understand how glaucoma is diagnosed.

History taking

Apart from acute angle-closure glaucoma, most forms of glaucoma are asymptomatic until very advanced optic nerve damage has occurred. A positive family history of glaucoma and myopia are important risk factors in the history.

Clinical examination

1 Visual acuity. Reduced by advanced chronic glaucoma damage or acute angle-closure glaucoma.

2 Ocular examination.

- Slit lamp examination for anterior segment abnormalities associated with glaucoma.
- Detailed assessment of optic disc. Ideally the optic disc is photographed (conventional or with 3D scanning laser ophthalmoscope) to enable detection of progression.

3 IOP measurement. Using Goldmann applanation tonometer. Measures force needed to flatten a defined area of cornea. This force corresponds to intraocular pressure (IOP, measured in mm of mercury). NB, low tension glaucoma has normal range IOP.

4 Visual field testing. Usually assessed with automated perimetry to allow efficient repeat testing to detect progression. Classic defect is arcuate scotoma.

5 Gonioscopy. Used to assess the anterior chamber angle. Can not be viewed directly so gonioprism lens is used—the optics of which allow visualization of the angle between the cornea and iris.

Glaucoma is diagnosed if a glaucomatous optic neuropathy (typical optic disc and field changes) is found to be present. Other parts of the examination help classify the glaucoma so appropriate treatment can be given.

> **TIP**
> Do not rely on IOP measurement alone for the diagnosis and monitoring of glaucoma as the IOP may be in the normal range, yet disc and field changes may be present.

Monitoring

Once a patient has been diagnosed and started on treatment, the same techniques are used at regular intervals to assess for progression. Finding the correct treatment to prevent progression is dependent on these same examination techniques.

Screening

Most forms of glaucoma are asymptomatic until very advanced optic nerve damage has occurred. Treatment at this stage is often too late, so glaucoma patients may be actively sought out from the community, i.e. screened. This is usually done by opticians, who assess IOP, visual fields and optic disc appearance. Two main groups of people are screened:

1 People with a family history of glaucoma, especially primary open-angle glaucoma.

2 All people over 40 will have IOP measured at a sight test.

If an abnormality suggestive of glaucoma is detected in this screening process, the person is referred to the hospital ophthalmology department.

Problems of glaucoma screening

- People are missed if they do not attend opticians.
- False positives are common because the initial assessment of field and disc is difficult.

> **WARNING**
> Some patients have low-tension glaucoma in which they have field loss and cupped discs with normal IOP.

KEY POINTS

- Glaucoma screening by opticians helps detect primary open-angle glaucoma.
- A family history of primary open-angle glaucoma is a risk factor for developing glaucoma.
- Automated visual field analysis is used to monitor visual field progression.

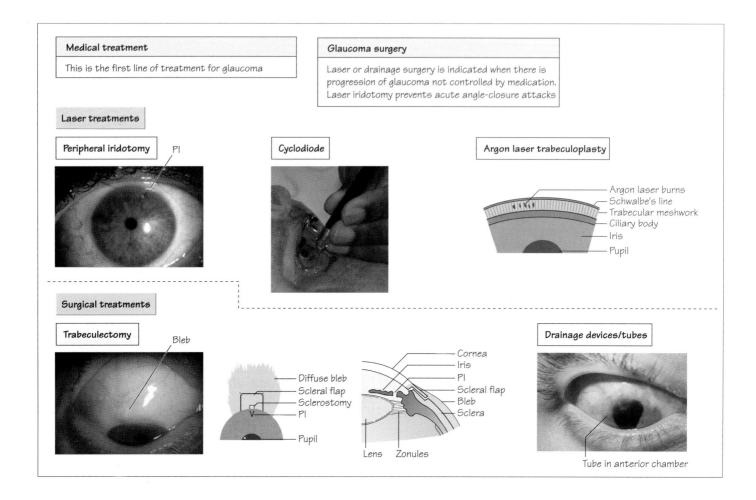

Medical treatment

This is the first line of treatment for glaucoma

Glaucoma surgery

Laser or drainage surgery is indicated when there is progression of glaucoma not controlled by medication. Laser iridotomy prevents acute angle-closure attacks

Laser treatments

Peripheral iridotomy — PI

Cyclodiode

Argon laser trabeculoplasty
- Argon laser burns
- Schwalbe's line
- Trabecular meshwork
- Ciliary body
- Iris
- Pupil

Surgical treatments

Trabeculectomy — Bleb

- Diffuse bleb
- Scleral flap
- Sclerostomy
- PI
- Pupil

- Cornea
- Iris
- PI
- Scleral flap
- Bleb
- Sclera

Lens   Zonules

Drainage devices/tubes

Tube in anterior chamber

Aims

1 Understand the aims of medical, laser and surgical treatment
2 Be familiar with the different classes of drugs used to treat chronic open-angle glaucoma.
3 Manage a case of acute angle-closure glaucoma (AACG).

Treatment goal

To preserve patient's sight throughout their lifetime with minimum side effects.
- **Treat to lower IOP.** This is the main aim of current glaucoma therapy.
- **Treat to increase ocular perfusion.** Prevent low blood pressure (nocturnal dips), treat vasospasm (calcium antagonists) and prevent arteriosclerosis.

Treatment options

1 Medical therapy.
2 Laser.
3 Surgery.

Medical therapy

Treatment is tailored to each patient's findings—intraocular pressure (IOP), visual field and optic disc appearance—and their type of glaucoma. Most patients with chronic open-angle glaucoma are treated medically and do not require surgery to drain the aqueous. The aim of medical treatment is to prevent progression of disc cupping or visual field defect.

Table of topical medical treatments

Class of agent	Method of action	Side effects	Examples (trade name)
Beta-blocker	Decreases aqueous humour production	Bradycardia/heart block Bronchoconstriction Depression Impotence	Timolol (Timoptol) Betaxolol (Betoptic) Carteolol (Teoptic) Levobunolol (Betagan)
Miotic (parasympathomimetic)	Increases outflow through trabecular meshwork	Blurred vision Headache Eye ache	Pilocarpine
Carbonic anhydrase inhibitor	Decreases aqueous humour production	Malaise Depression Metallic taste	Dorzolamide (Trusopt) Brinzolamide (Azopt) Acetazolamide (Diamox), oral and i.v.
Alpha-1 agonist	Decreases aqueous production and increases uveoscleral outflow	Allergy Dry mouth Fatigue	Brimonidine (Alphagan) Apraclonidine (Iopidine)
Prostaglandin agonist	Increases uveoscleral outflow	Increased iris pigment Eyelash growth Macular oedema	Latanoprost (Xalatan) Travoprost (Travatan)
Docosanoid	Increases uveoscleral outflow	Allergy Nausea Nasal congestion	Unoprostone (Rescula)
Prostamide	Increases uveoscleral outflow	Allergy	Bimatoprost (Lumigan)
Adrenergic agonist	Increases uveoscleral outflow	Rarely used now	Epinephrine (Eppy) Dipivinyl epinephrine (Propine)

Laser treatment

• **Peripheral iridotomy.** Procedure of choice to prevent angle-closure glaucoma or after an acute attack has been broken with medical treatment. A YAG laser hole in the iris allows aqueous flow from posterior to anterior chamber.
• **Cyclodestruction.** Diode laser (usually) to ciliary body to reduce aqueous production.
• **Argon laser trabeculoplasty.** Laser to trabecular meshwork to increase aqueous outflow.

Surgical treatment

• **Peripheral iridectomy.** Used in AACG when laser is not possible.
• **Trabeculectomy.** Standard glaucoma surgery to filter aqueous from anterior chamber to subconjunctival space, used most commonly for open-angle glaucoma. Antimetabolites such as 5-fluorouracil and mitomycin C are used to modulate conjunctival healing and improve success rates. Risks include cataract, hypotony, infection and bleb leakage.

Other surgical techniques

• **Drainage devices/tubes.** Silicone tube inserted into anterior chamber and connected to subconjunctival silicone chamber to drain aqueous. Used when trabeculectomy may fail, for instance in congenital glaucoma and some of the secondary glaucomas.
• **Deep sclerectomy.** Section of sclera and roof of Schlemm's canal are excised. No penetration into anterior chamber so less complications than trabeculectomy, but less IOP control.
• **Viscocanalostomy.** Deep sclerectomy with additional mechanical opening of Schlemm's canal by injecting high viscosity fluid.

WARNING
Acute angle-closure glaucoma (AACG) is an ophthalmic emergency.

Treatment of AACG

AACG requires medical, laser and surgical treatment. Immediate treatment is medical to reduce the IOP and to break the attack of angle closure.

• Intravenous carbonic anhydrase inhibitor (**acetazolamide 500 mg**) is used to halt the production of aqueous fluid.
• Oral acetazolamide may also be needed for up to 24 h.
• Pilocarpine may be needed to break the attack, but is not used intensively.
• Other topical agents will also help reduce the IOP (**timolol** or **iopidine**).
• To prevent further attacks: pilocarpine drops (2–4%) are used (not intensively) in both eyes to constrict the pupil as a temporary measure. Bilateral laser iridotomies (and occasionally surgical irridectomy) must then be performed as a permanent prevention.
• Rarely, trabeculectomy is required.

KEY POINTS
• Most primary open-angle glaucoma patients are treated medically, e.g. with topical beta-blockers.
• Trabeculectomy lowers the IOP by draining aqueous into a small subconjunctival bleb from where the fluid is reabsorbed.
• Surgery is indicated for disease progression in primary open-angle glaucoma.

39 Retinal detachment

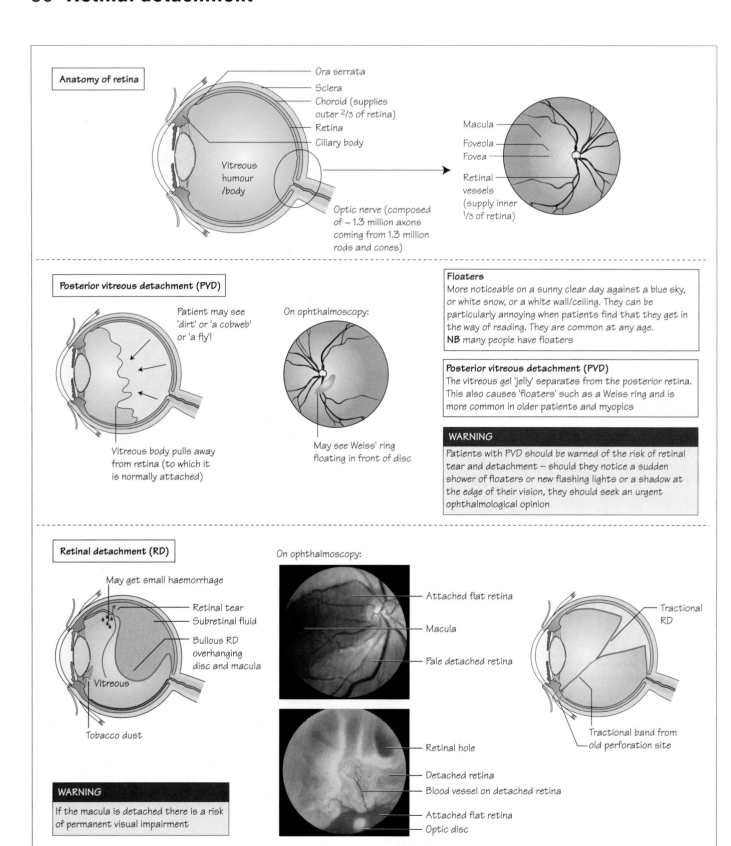

Anatomy of retina

Ora serrata
Sclera
Choroid (supplies outer 2/3 of retina)
Retina
Ciliary body

Vitreous humour /body

Optic nerve (composed of ~ 1.3 million axons coming from 1.3 million rods and cones)

Macula
Foveola
Fovea
Retinal vessels (supply inner 1/3 of retina)

Posterior vitreous detachment (PVD)

Patient may see 'dirt' or 'a cobweb' or 'a fly'!

Vitreous body pulls away from retina (to which it is normally attached)

On ophthalmoscopy:

May see Weiss' ring floating in front of disc

Floaters
More noticeable on a sunny clear day against a blue sky, or white snow, or a white wall/ceiling. They can be particularly annoying when patients find that they get in the way of reading. They are common at any age.
NB many people have floaters

Posterior vitreous detachment (PVD)
The vitreous gel 'jelly' separates from the posterior retina. This also causes 'floaters' such as a Weiss ring and is more common in older patients and myopics

WARNING
Patients with PVD should be warned of the risk of retinal tear and detachment – should they notice a sudden shower of floaters or new flashing lights or a shadow at the edge of their vision, they should seek an urgent ophthalmological opinion

Retinal detachment (RD)

May get small haemorrhage

Retinal tear
Subretinal fluid
Bullous RD overhanging disc and macula

Vitreous

Tobacco dust

On ophthalmoscopy:

Attached flat retina
Macula
Pale detached retina

Retinal hole
Detached retina
Blood vessel on detached retina
Attached flat retina
Optic disc

Tractional RD

Tractional band from old perforation site

WARNING
If the macula is detached there is a risk of permanent visual impairment

Aims

1 Understand significance of eye floaters.
2 Types of retinal detachment.
3 Principles of managing a retinal tear.

Posterior vitreous detachment (PVD)

A PVD is when the posterior aspect of the vitreous body pulls away or separates from the retina and collapses towards the vitreous base. Noticed as a floating cobweb, ring or tadpole, which moves with eye movement.

Aetiology

• Trauma to the eye or head.
• Spontaneous—especially in myopic eyes. Onset can be gradual or more acute, and is due to degeneration of the vitreous gel.

Symptoms

• Photopsia (i.e. flashing lights) results from physical traction of the retina—not necessarily indicating a retinal tear. The flashing lights are more noticeable in dim lighting.
• Floaters result from a small amount of haemorrhage which may occur, or the collapsed vitreous which casts a shadow on the retina. A ring shape (Weiss' ring) may be seen or cobwebs or a tadpole shape.

Natural history of floaters

The majority of floaters from PVD are self-limiting, setting as occasional floaters and becoming less noticeable. Only a small proportion of patients develop a retinal tear.

Complications

In up to 15% of patients who present with an **acute symptomatic PVD** the detaching vitreous pulls a hole in the retina, which can lead to a rhegmatogenous retinal detachment.

Management

• Full retinal assessment is needed to rule out a retinal tear—examine through dilated pupils. The periphery of the retina can be seen on the slit lamp using a three-mirror contact lens. Indirect ophthalmoscopy with scleral indentation is the best method of mapping the retinal detachment and location of the retinal tear.
• If a simple retinal tear is present with minimal or no subretinal fluid—use laser treatment to seal the tear and to prevent retinal detachment.
• No tear—reassurance only, no treatment is required.

Retinal detachment (RD)

• An RD occurs when the retina is separated from the retinal pigment epithelium (RPE) by fluid (this fluid is known as subretinal fluid or SRF).
• Once the retina has been separated from its main blood supply, the photoreceptors slowly begin to degenerate, becoming non-functional by 6 weeks.
• It is therefore essential that once an RD has been diagnosed, that it is surgically reattached as soon as possible in order to regain vision.
• If the macula is detached (off) surgery is urgent.

Aetiology

• A full thickness tear in the retina, which may result from a spontaneous PVD or may occur as a result of trauma, allows liquid vitreous to enter the space between the retina and the RPE. This type of RD is known as a **rhegmatogenous retinal detachment**. Individuals with high myopia are at increased risk of this type of RD.
• Some inflammatory and neoplastic conditions can lead to serous exudation from leaky blood vessels beneath the retina in the absence of a retinal break or hole, this is referred to as an **exudative retinal detachment**.
• Fibrous or vascular membranes growing abnormally in the vitreous (e.g. in patients with diabetes or who have had a penetrating eye injury) can contract and pull the retina away from the RPE. This is known as a **tractional retinal detachment**.
• A tumour such as a malignant melanoma originating in the choroid behind the retina can elevate the retina, causing a **solid retinal detachment**. This can metastasize and needs urgent treatment.

Symptoms

Rhegmatogenous RD presents with:
• Photopsia ± floaters.
• Followed by gradual blurring or loss of vision, which may start off as a shadow in the peripheral visual field. As the SRF spreads to involve the macula, the vision becomes very blurred.
• Other types of RD present with reduced vision.

Signs

• Visual acuity may appear normal when macula on.
• Reduced visual acuity may be due to macular SRF or may result from a bullous RD falling in front of the macula.
• On slit lamp examination, 'tobacco dust' may be visible in the anterior vitreous (these are red blood cells and/or RPE cells that have migrated into the vitreous from the tear).
• Intraocular pressure may be reduced.
• Detached retina on fundoscopy—indirect ophthalmoscopy with scleral indentation is the preferred method of viewing this. A three-mirror contact lens at the slit lamp can be used if a retinal tear is likely to require laser treatment and not full surgery.

Complications

• If the RD involves the macular area, the chance of regaining vision is very much reduced.
• Recurrent RD carries the risk of subretinal membrane and secondary tractional detachment.

Management

• Rhegmatogenous RD—use reattachment surgery: laser, cryotherapy plus explant or internal surgery with vitrectomy.
• Exudative and solid RD—establish and treat the cause.
• Tractional RD—relieve traction by vitreoretinal surgery.

KEY POINTS

• PVD results in floaters and there *may* be a retinal tear.
• Subretinal fluid gets under the retina through a tear and lifts the sensory retina off the retinal pigment epithelium, causing a detachment.
• Some RDs do not have tears but are exudative, tractional or solid in origin.

40 Retinal and choroidal anatomy and imaging

Knowledge of retinal anatomy and physiology is vital to interpret retinal images

Anatomy

Choroid: fenestrated capillary-rich layer which supplies oxygen and micronutrients to the retinal pigment epithelium and the outer third of the neurosensory retina. The capillary layer is the choriocapillaris

Retinal pigment epithelium (RPE): monolayer of pigmented cells between the neurosensory retina and Bruch's membrane. Tight junctions exclude large molecules and form the outer part of the blood retinal barrier

Bruch's membrane: an acellular layer between the choroid and RPE, which does not form a significant part of the blood retinal barrier

Neurosensory retina: includes photoreceptors, ganglion cells and their axons (nerve fibre layer), other neurons (e.g. bipolar cells) and glial cells (e.g. Müller cells)

Retinal arteries, capillaries and veins: non-fenestrated vessels forming the inner blood retinal barrier

Foveal avascular zone: approximately 0.045 mm zone in which retinal capillaries are absent

Fovea
Foveola
Inner limiting membrane
Retinal vessels
Ganglion cell layer
Layer of intermediary neurons
Photoreceptor layer
Cones only
Cones, some rods
Rods and cones
Retinal pigment epithelium
Bruch's membrane
Choriocapillaris

Retina
Choroid
Sclera

Human methylmethacrylate vascular cast

Inner choriocapillaris surface — large surface area for nutrient exchange to the outer retina

Cross section of choroid showing flattened choriocapillary sheet and outer larger choroidal blood vessels

Flat sheet chorio-capillaris

Copyright J Olver

Copyright J Olver

Retinal pigment epithelium cells
Bruch's membrane
Choriocapillaris
Intermediate-sized choroidal vessels
Outer larger choroidal vessels
Choroid

Fluorescein photography filters

Exciter filter 490 mm
Barrier filter 515 mm
Energy
Absorption spectrum
Emission spectrum
400 500 600
Wavelength (nm)

Topography of the posterior pole and retina

area centralis
Posterior pole
d = 5–6 mm
Optic disc
d = 1.5mm
fovea
Macula
d = 1.5 mm
foveola
Fovea
d = 0.35 mm

- Posterior pole area centralis (5–6 mm)
- Macula fovea (1.5 mm)
- Fovea foveola (350 ∝m)

Indiocyanine green photography filters

Exciter filter 795 mm
Barrier filter 830 mm
Energy
Absorption spectrum
Emission spectrum
700 800 900
Wavelength (nm)

Retinopathy pre-laser treatment

Normal left macula in same eye seen with i) fluorescein and ii) indocyanine green

Disc new vessels

Fluorescein angiogram in a diabetic showing leaking 'new vessels elsewhere'

FAZ

i) Retinal vessels imaged with fluorescein angiogram showing loss of capillary network at foveal avascular zone (FAZ)

ii) Choroidal vessels imaged. Indocyanine green angiogram (ICGA) showing rich choroidal blood supply at macula

Fundus fluorescein angiogram of a left eye with gross myopia and consequent chorioretinal degeneration and atrophy

Aims

1 Know the anatomy of the choroid and retina.
2 Identify the main priorities of medical retinal disease.
3 Methods of retinal imaging and appropriate use of a particular imaging system.
4 Understand the need for more than one modality of imaging.

Medical retinal disease priorities

Diabetic retinopathy and age-related macular degeneration are the main priorities in medical retina in terms of socioeconomic health care burden (see Chapter 3) but vascular occlusions occur commonly with age particularly in association with systemic disease. The inherited retinal dystrophies affect 1 in 4000 of the population—young and old. The management of medical retinal disease has been revolutionized as a result of developments in retinal imaging, the advent of molecular genetics and new treatment modalities.

Retinal imaging modalities, together with psychophysical and electrophysiological evaluation, are very valuable in diagnosing disorders of the retina, retinal pigment epithelium (RPE) and choroid.

Imaging

A fundus camera can be used to document baseline retinal findings, track disease progression, screening (e.g. for diabetic retinopathy) and clinical studies.
- A fundus camera ensures high resolution, high quality images.
- Colour fundus photography, fluorescein and indocyanine green angiography are used to image the retina and surrounding structures.
- Digital images allow rapid diagnosis and review, and are electronically transferred; they are useful for telemedicine.

Dyes used in imaging

Fluorescein. Sodium fluorescein is an orange dye that is excited by a blue light to emit a yellow-green light. It is a small molecule, only 80% bound to blood proteins, which diffuses freely through the choriocapillaris, Bruch's membrane, optic nerve and sclera.

Indocyanine green (ICG). This is a green dye, which when excited by a near infrared light emits a near infrared light. It is almost 100% protein bound so it only leaks slowly through the fenestrated capillaries of the choriocapillaris.

Fundus fluorescein angiogram (FFA)

This is a sequence of fundus images taken immediately after sodium fluorescein dye is injected into a peripheral vein. The fundus is illuminated by a blue light causing the fluorescein molecules to fluoresce in the yellow-green spectrum. Barrier filters block reflected blue light so that only yellow-green (i.e. fluorescent) light is transmitted to the film or digital camera. A detailed 3D view of the retina and of the level of fluorescence can be achieved by using a stereoscopic viewing device or computer software. Good for viewing retinal detail.

Indocyanine green angiography (ICGA)

Near infrared fluorescence is recorded with infrared film or more commonly with a digital camera, after the injection of ICG into a peripheral vein. Light of this wavelength has better penetration of red or brown pigments (e.g. melanin in RPE cells or subretinal blood). ICGA is useful in investigating choroidal disease, e.g. choroidal neovascularization and choroidal tumours.

Confocal scanning laser ophthalmoscope (SLO)

A fundus camera using a low-power scanning laser for illumination at different focal planes in the retina to produce **tomographic images**.

Optical coherence tomography (OCT)

Non-invasive diagnostic imaging analogous to an ultrasound B scan except that light and not sound is used; a higher resolution is therefore obtainable. A highly coherent light source is used to scan the retina and produces high-resolution, cross-sectional and 3D images. Used for assessing retinal thickness, retinal oedema and optic nerve head imaging in glaucoma.

Terms used when describing fluorescein angiograms

Hyperfluorescence: Increased fluorescence relative to other structures seen as black on white if negative film is used and white on black with digital photography.
Hypofluorescence: Reduced fluorescence relative to other structures, e.g. due to blocked fluorescence or decreased vascular perfusion.
Window defect: Increased choroidal fluorescence seen through a window of attenuated RPE, e.g. geographic atrophy or laser scars.
Blocked fluorescence: Masking of fluorescence by opacity anterior to it, e.g. subretinal haemorrhage.
Fluorescein leakage: Characteristic of conditions in which the outer (RPE) or inner (retinal vasculature) blood–retinal barrier is disrupted.
Autofluorescence: Fluorescence occurring without the injection of fluorescein dye.

Side effects of fluorescein and indocyanine green

		Fluorescein	Indocyanine green (ICG)
Contraindications			
	Absolute	Fluorescein allergy History of severe allergies	ICG, iodine or shellfish allergy History of severe allergies
	Relative	Asthma Ischaemic heart disease Previous allergic reaction Renal failure (use lower dose)	Asthma Ischaemic heart disease Previous allergic reaction Liver failure
Adverse effects		Skin discolouration Nausea 3–5% Allergy 0.5–1%	Mild to moderate 0.35% (e.g. hypotension) Severe 0.05% (e.g. anaphylaxis)
Excretion		Liver and kidneys	Liver

KEY POINTS

- Fluorescein angiography provides fine detail of the retinal structures and vessels.
- Indocyanine green provides information about the choroidal vessels.
- There are potential side effects or complications of these dyes.

Microanatomy

Photoreceptors: Rods: for vision in dim light (shades of black and white) and motion vision. Cones: for vision in bright light (high resolution and colour). Rods predominate outside the fovea, cones are most dense at the fovea. **Retinal Pigment Epithelium (RPE):** Single layer of cells with an important role in the turnover and support of photoreceptor outer-segments and formation of photosensitive pigments. Forms the **blood-retinal barrier.** **Bruch's Membrane:** Separates the RPE from choriocapillaris. See Chapter 40

Definitions

Dystrophy: Inherited disorder
Photophobia: Painful sensation in bright light
Nyctalopia: Poor or lack of vision in the dark
Phenotype: Clinical characterization including symptoms (e.g. photophobia, nyctalopia), fundus appearance and functional assessment

Inherited retinal dystrophies

A. Peripheral dystrophies – affect peripheral vision and vision in low light levels, e.g. retinitis pigmentosa, choroideraemia and Leber's congenital amaurosis
Retinitis pigmentosa (RP) varies in severity, mode of inheritance, age at onset, progression and phenotype. Inheritance patterns include: autosomal dominant (AD), autosomal recessive (AR), X-linked (Xl). Mitochondrial and syndromic retinopathy are also described

B. Central dystrophies – affect the macular region. Early onset central visual difficulties with photophobia, loss of detailed vision and colour vision defects, e.g. cone dystrophies, macular dystrophies including Best disease, Stargardt/fundus flavimaculatus, Sorsby, Bull's eye, Dominant drusen (Doyne honeycombe) dystrophy

C. Mixed dystropies – Cone–rods affected with loss of central and peripheral vision

D. Syndromal – e.g. AR Usher syndrome with hearing loss and RP

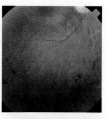

Peripheral dystrophy: Retinitis pigmentosa with intra retinal mid peripheral bone spicule pigmentation

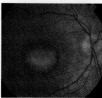

Central dystrophy: Best dystrophy

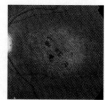

Mixed dystrophy: cone rod

Classification of age related macular degeneration (AMD)

ARM

Histopathology and colour fundus picture of soft confluent Drusen at macula
Courtesy of Victor Chong

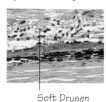
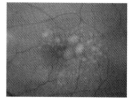

Soft Drusen

AMD

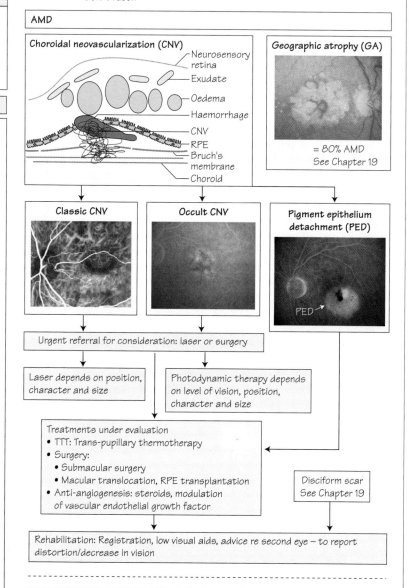

Choroidal neovascularization (CNV)
- Neurosensory retina
- Exudate
- Oedema
- Haemorrhage
- CNV
- RPE
- Bruch's membrane
- Choroid

Geographic atrophy (GA)

= 80% AMD
See Chapter 19

Classic CNV

Occult CNV

Pigment epithelium detachment (PED)

PED→

Urgent referral for consideration: laser or surgery

Laser depends on position, character and size

Photodynamic therapy depends on level of vision, position, character and size

Treatments under evaluation
- TTT: Trans-pupillary thermotherapy
- Surgery:
  - Submacular surgery
  - Macular translocation, RPE transplantation
- Anti-angiogenesis: steroids, modulation of vascular endothelial growth factor

Disciform scar
See Chapter 19

Rehabilitation: Registration, low visual aids, advice re second eye – to report distortion/decrease in vision

Educate AMD patient to report if decrease or distortion in vision. Consider vitamin supplementation: Age Related Eye Disease Study recommendations. See Amsler chart, Chapter 7

Aims

1 Types of inherited retinal degeneration.
2 Know the significance of early central visual symptoms and prompt referral for possible early treatment of neovascular age-related macular degeneration (AMD).
3 Treatment options and importance of low-vision aids and social support in both inherited retinal degeneration and AMD.

Skills to obtain

Use the ophthalmoscope to learn to recognize retinitis pigmentosa and AMD.

Inherited retinal dystrophies

A large number of disorders with progressive retinal degeneration which are variable in severity, age of onset and may have distinguishing phenotypic and functional features. The term retinitis pigmentosa is used to describe peripheral dystrophies, but the latter term covers a spectrum of inherited progressive retinal degenerations. Features include night blindness, progressive visual field loss, reduced or non-recordable electroretinograms and characteristic pigmentary retinal degenerative changes in 1 in 4000.

Classification of these disorders is enhanced by knowledge of the inheritance pattern, causative gene(s) and mutation(s) if known, and more sophisticated phenotypic characterization including psychophysics and electrophysiology.

Age-related macular degeneration

- Commonest cause of blindness in the elderly population.
- Approximately 2% of over 65 year olds are registered blind in one or both eyes from AMD in the UK.
  - Geographic atrophy accounts for approximately 80%.
  - Treatment options are limited and are mainly targeted at neovascular AMD using laser photocoagulation or photodynamic therapy. Anti-angiogenesis therapies are being evaluated.
  - Early symptoms require prompt referral for evaluation and possible treatment of choroidal neovascularization (CNV). See Chapter 7, Amsler chart.

Definitions

- **Age-related maculopathy (ARM)**: Disorder of the macular area most often occurring after 50 years of age, characterized by Drusen ± changes in the retinal pigment epithelium (RPE).
- **Age-related macular degeneration (AMD)**: Late stages of ARM that lead to progressive central vision loss. Includes: geographic atrophy of the RPE and subsequently photoreceptor cell loss, CNV, pigment epithelial detachment, haemorrhages, exudates and scar tissue.
- **Drusen**: Yellowish deposits external to the neuroretina and RPE. May be well defined and small (hard) or ill defined (soft). Drusen may be discrete or confluent and are hallmarks of age-related change found at the level of Bruch's membrane.
- **Geographic atrophy (GA)**: Demarcated zones of apparent RPE atrophy. Associated with Drusen. Gradual central vision loss.
- **Choroidal neovascularization (CNV)**: Abnormal new blood vessels that arise from the choroid and proliferate with subsequent fibrous tissue. Often not identifiable on ophthalmoscopy but may be visualized using FFA.
- **Disciform scar**: Subretinal fibrovascular scar. Usually part of the healing response following CNV. Permanent vision loss occurs as the outer retina (including photoreceptors) becomes atrophic or replaced by fibrous scar tissue.

- **Pigment epithelial detachment (PED)**: Accumulation of oedema ± blood beneath the RPE. An underlying CNV is commonly present in older patients.
- **Retinal oedema and exudate**: Leakage of serum into and behind the retina from CNV. Lipid components not easily removed by macrophages accumulate, often at the edge of the oedema, as characteristic yellowish lesions.

Pathology

- **RPE.** Accumulation of photoreceptor, outer-segment waste products and vesicular granular material. GA may be due to reduced metabolic exchange between the choroid and RPE.
- **Bruch's membrane.** Focal and diffuse thickening with age. Accumulation of Drusen and presumed degrade collagen material from the RPE.
- **Choroid.** Neovascularization arises from the capillary layer of choroid. Photoreceptor atrophy and scarring begins early in neovascularization, even without haemorrhage.

Risk factors for AMD

- Genetic and environmental are implicated.
- Cigarette smoking is a known risk factor.
- Vascular disease, hypertension and light exposure are associated with AMD but are not risk factors.
- Supplementation with extra carotenoids, certain vitamins and antioxidants may be associated with a decreased risk of developing AMD in certain types of ARM/AMD.

Diagnosis and assessment

- Recent symptoms of central distortion/blurring raise the possibility of neovascular AMD.
- An Amsler chart (p. 20) is useful in evaluating central vision.
- Gradual decline, however, suggests GA.
- *Dilated fundus examination and FFA is essential in order to identify treatable CNV.*

Treatment

- Various types of laser, including photodynamic therapy for neovascular AMD.
- 90% of AMD is **untreatable**. GA or neovascular AMD with occult subfoveal CNV often results in significant scarring and/or haemorrhage. New therapies are undergoing evaluation.

Rehabilitation

Blind/partially sighted registration
- Financial allowance.
- Talking books/clocks.
- Home visit by low-vision therapist to assess disability.
- Initiate community care, Social and/or voluntary services.
- Contact with self-help groups.

Low-vision aids (see Chapter 9)
- **Optical aids**: magnifiers, telescopes.
- **Non-optical aids**: lighting, large print books/bank statements.
- **Electronic aids**: closed circuit television (CCTV).

KEY POINTS

- Inherited retinal degenerations common, but no therapy available.
- AMD is the leading cause of blindness in industrialized countries.
- Sudden-onset central distortion/blurring may represent treatable CNV.

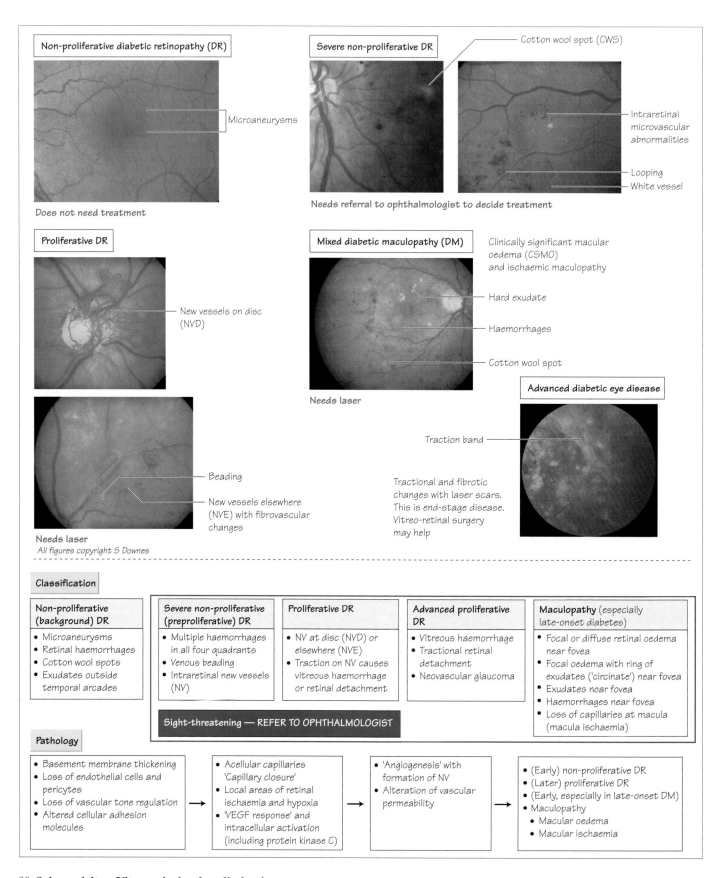

Non-proliferative diabetic retinopathy (DR)

Microaneurysms

Does not need treatment

Severe non-proliferative DR

Cotton wool spot (CWS)

Intraretinal microvascular abnormalities

Looping

White vessel

Needs referral to ophthalmologist to decide treatment

Proliferative DR

New vessels on disc (NVD)

Beading

New vessels elsewhere (NVE) with fibrovascular changes

Needs laser

All figures copyright S Downes

Mixed diabetic maculopathy (DM)

Clinically significant macular oedema (CSMO) and ischaemic maculopathy

Hard exudate

Haemorrhages

Cotton wool spot

Needs laser

Advanced diabetic eye disease

Traction band

Tractional and fibrotic changes with laser scars. This is end-stage disease. Vitreo-retinal surgery may help

Classification

Non-proliferative (background) DR	Severe non-proliferative (preproliferative) DR	Proliferative DR	Advanced proliferative DR	Maculopathy (especially late-onset diabetes)
• Microaneurysms • Retinal haemorrhages • Cotton wool spots • Exudates outside temporal arcades	• Multiple haemorrhages in all four quadrants • Venous beading • Intraretinal new vessels (NV)	• NV at disc (NVD) or elsewhere (NVE) • Traction on NV causes vitreous haemorrhage or retinal detachment	• Vitreous haemorrhage • Tractional retinal detachment • Neovascular glaucoma	• Focal or diffuse retinal oedema near fovea • Focal oedema with ring of exudates ('circinate') near fovea • Exudates near fovea • Haemorrhages near fovea • Loss of capillaries at macula (macula ischaemia)

Sight-threatening — REFER TO OPHTHALMOLOGIST

Pathology

• Basement membrane thickening
• Loss of endothelial cells and pericytes
• Loss of vascular tone regulation
• Altered cellular adhesion molecules
	→ • Acellular capillaries 'Capillary closure'
	• Local areas of retinal ischaemia and hypoxia
	• 'VEGF response' and intracellular activation (including protein kinase C)
		→ • 'Angiogenesis' with formation of NV
		• Alteration of vascular permeability
			→ • (Early) non-proliferative DR
			• (Later) proliferative DR
			• (Early, especially in late-onset DM)
			• Maculopathy
			  • Macular oedema
			  • Macular ischaemia

Aims

1 Learn the classification of diabetic retinopathy (DR) and its pathogenesis.

2 Be aware of contributory risk factors to severity of retinopathy (e.g. duration of diabetes, pregnancy, blood pressure).

3 Understand the importance of DR screening.

• DR is the major cause of poor vision in the working population in the UK, Ireland, USA, Australia and the Indian subcontinent. The annual incidence of blindness from DR varies between 0.02% and 1%.

• Alterations in different biochemical pathways as a result of diabetes have been implicated in the development of the microvasculature abnormalities that are seen in DR.

• An international standard classification of DR is essential for guidelines in screening, treatment protocols and research.

Definitions

Microaneurysms: Outpouching of retinal capillaries. May bleed, leak or become occluded.

Cotton wool spot: Microinfarct of the retinal nerve fibre layer (NFL) causing a localized swelling of the NFL axon (non-specific indicator of retinal ischaemia).

Retinal oedema and exudate: Leakage of serum into the neural retina due to vessel wall damage. Lipid components that are not easily removed by macrophages accumulate, often at the edge of the oedema, as characteristic yellowish lesions.

Venous beading: Venous irregularities, 'sausaging' and engorgement. Sign of retinal ischaemia and powerful predictor of conversion to proliferative retinopathy.

Retinal neovascularization/new vessels: Fragile new vessels grow outside the retina along the posterior surface of the vitreous. Changes in bloodflow or traction on the new vessels, including posterior vitreous detachment, may cause them to haemorrhage into the vitreous cavity (vitreous haemorrhage).

Pathology

Microvasculature changes causing ischaemia

• Basement membrane thickening, endothelial cell damage and loss, and increased platelet adhesiveness lead to narrowing of the retinal vessels and hence **ischaemia**.

Ischaemia is manifest as: cotton wool spots, deep retinal haemorrhages, venous beading and new vessel formation/ neovascularization (whose growth is induced by the release of angiogenic cytokines from the ischaemic retina).

• If new vessels grow at the optic disc they are referred to as **NVD**.

• If new vessels grow at any other location they are described as new vessels elsewhere (**NVE**).

The new vessels are a response to hypoxia and ischaemia in an attempt to increase the oxygen supply to the retina. However, these vessels are weak and friable and bleed easily casing vitreous haemorrhage. They may also cause traction on the retina resulting in tractional retinal detachment.

Microvascular changes resulting in leaking vessels

• Endothelial cell loss, pericyte loss of vascular tone result in *increased permeability* of the retinal vessels and hence *exudation* of blood and blood products into the retina.

• Blot and dot haemorrhages, hard exudates and diffuse oedema are seen.

• These changes can also lead to localized vessel wall weakness and microaneurysm formation. These microaneurysms leak and exudates form in a circle around the aneurysm—'circinate exudates'.

Screening

• DR is the leading cause of blindness in the working population in the UK.

• Twenty-five per cent of diabetics develop DR; 10–13% of diabetics have sight-threatening DR.

• Prevalence of DR increases with duration of diabetes.

• Natural history of DR is known.

• Early treatment is effective in preventing visual impairment.

• An effective screening service requires effective recall of eligible patients, 80% sensitivity, 95% specificity and quality assurance.

• Digital photographic screening is the preferred method.

• Detection of any DR should direct attention towards improving blood pressure and glycaemic control.

KEY POINTS

• DR is the leading cause of blindness in the working population of the developed world.

• Screening and early treatment can prevent vision loss.

• Uncontrolled hypertension makes DR worse.

43 Diabetic retinopathy treatment

Treatment options

Blood pressure, lipid and glycaemic control

- Reduce progression and severity of diabetic retinopathy (DR)
- Reduce need for laser

Panretinal photocoagulation (PRP) laser

- Laser (usually argon)
- Indicated for proliferative DR to reduce risk of vision loss due to vitreous haemorrhage or tractional retinal detachment

Macular laser

- Focal or grid pattern
- Encourages absorption of oedema

Vitrectomy

Aims: to
- Clear vitreous haemorrhage
- Allow further PRP laser
- Relieve retinal traction and repair retinal detachment
- Treat diffuse macula oedema due to vitreous traction

In the UK and Ireland, the National Framework for Diabetes aims to raise the standards for diabetic care including DR, and reduce blindness from DR

Proliferative diabetic retinopathy (DR)

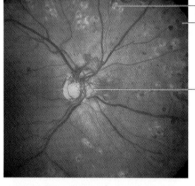

— Panretinal photocoagulation

— New vessels on disc (NVD)

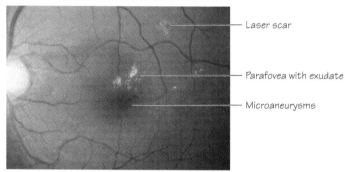

— Panretinal photocoagulation

— New vessels elsewhere (NVE) — still proliferative and undergoing more laser

Needs more laser

Clinically significant macular oedema (CSMO)

— Laser scar

— Parafovea with exudate

— Microaneurysms

Needs more laser

Treated CSMO

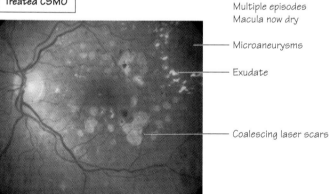

Multiple episodes Macula now dry

— Microaneurysms

— Exudate

— Coalescing laser scars

Needs gentle laser burns

DR treatment options

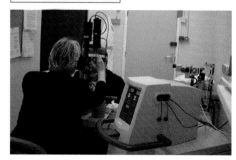

(a)

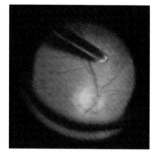

(b)

Good diabetic, blood pressure and lipid control. Antiangiogenesis agents under evaluation. Current therapies include (a) laser and (b) vitrectomy surgery

Aims

1 Be aware of the treatment options in diabetic retinopathy (DR).
2 Be able to explain about laser treatment to the patient.

- **Blood pressure, lipid and glycaemic control:**
  —reduces the progression and severity of DR;
  —reduces the need for laser treatment.
- Patients should also be advised not to smoke as this contributes to vascular damage.
- Any underlying anaemia should be treated.

> **TIP**
> Early treatment = better vision.

Treatment options

The commonest treatment for DR is laser photocoagulation—either panretinal, or focal laser or grid laser to the macula. DR often requires multiple treatments.

Panretinal photocoagulation (PRP)

- Indicated for proliferative DR to reduce the risk of vision loss due to vitreous haemorrhage or tractional retinal detachment.
- An argon laser is used to produce 1500–3000 tiny burns in the peripheral retina, sparing the macula, papillomacular bundle and optic nerve head. This causes regression of new vessels at the optic disc (NVD) and new vessels elsewhere (NVE).
- The patient will have reduced peripheral and night vision post PRP.
- PRP is performed in the out-patient clinic using a laser attached to a slit lamp. The treatment requires topical anaesthesia as a special contact lens is used to apply the laser burns.
- Depending on the patient's ability to tolerate the treatment and the amount of burns required, the laser is applied over a number of sessions.

- Once adequate laser has been applied, the abnormal vessels will regress in about 8 weeks.

Macular laser

- **Focal laser** is used to destroy microaneurysms that are leaking exudate into the macular area. After the aneurysm has been treated the exudates will resorb.
- **Grid laser** is used to treat non-ischaemic diffuse macular oedema. The entire macula, excluding the fovea, is treated with very tiny low-powered laser in order to encourage absorption of oedema.
- Patients must be warned that macular laser treatment is used to prevent vision getting worse, and does not always improve visual acuity. Some patients notice a scotoma after macular laser treatment.

Vitrectomy

This is a specialized procedure whereby the vitreous is removed via a trans-pars plana incision, hence the term trans-pars plana vitrectomy (TPPV). TPPV is carried out by a vitreoretinal surgeon, usually under general anaesthesia.

Indications
- To clear vitreous haemorrhage—this allows the surgeon to visualize the retina and apply further PRP laser.
- To relieve retinal traction and repair retinal detachment.
- To treat diffuse macula oedema due to vitreous traction.

> **KEY POINTS**
> - Tight blood pressure, lipid and glycaemic control reduces the progression and severity of DR and the need for laser treatment.
> - PRP is the treatment for proliferative DR.
> - Focal laser is used to treat leaking microaneurysms at the macula, that are threatening vision.

The central retinal vein drains all the layers of the retina and the optic nerve head anterior to the lamina cribosa. When it is occluded, there is marked venous engorgement and leakage with retinal oedema, ischaemia and haemorrhage

Anatomy

Central retinal vein (CRV) course at optic nerve head

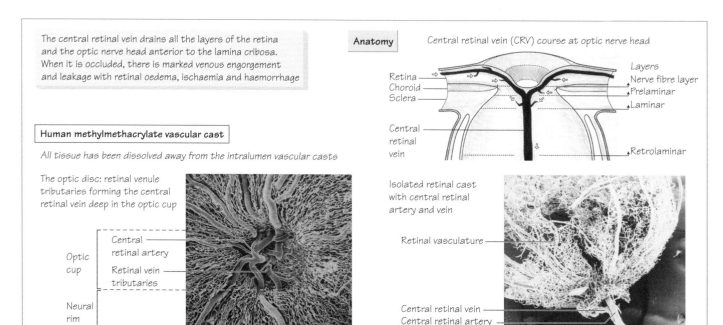

Retina
Choroid
Sclera

Central retinal vein

Layers
Nerve fibre layer
Prelaminar
Laminar
Retrolaminar

Human methylmethacrylate vascular cast

All tissue has been dissolved away from the intralumen vascular casts

The optic disc: retinal venule tributaries forming the central retinal vein deep in the optic cup

Optic cup

Central retinal artery

Retinal vein tributaries

Neural rim

Copyright J Olver

Isolated retinal cast with central retinal artery and vein

Retinal vasculature

Central retinal vein
Central retinal artery

Copyright J Olver

Central retinal vein occlusion (CRVO) (left eye)

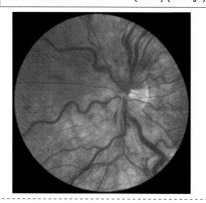

Neovascular glaucoma – iris new vessels and pathology

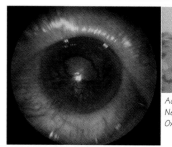

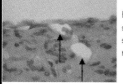

Histopathology of iris surface with arrows showing iris neovascularization

Acknowledgements to Dr Brendon McDonald, Neuropathologist, Oxford Radcliffe Infirmary, Oxford for the histopathology slide

Rubeosis iridis: (iris neovascularization) – end-stage disease

Branch retinal vein occlusion (BRVO)

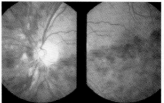

Affecting three quadrants (left eye)

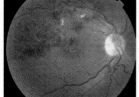

Affecting one quadrant (right eye)

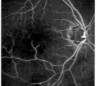

Fluorescein angiogram of branch vein occlusion

Hypertensive retinopathy

- Usually asymptomatic and bilateral
- Can have BRVO or CRVO
- Range of features from generalized retinal arteriolar narrowing, cotton wool spots, exudates, arteriovenous crossing changes, flame-shaped haemorrhages, to optic nerve head swelling

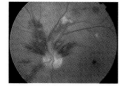

Retinal flame haemorrhages

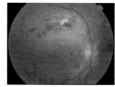

BRVO and silver wiring

Medical associations with retinal vein occlusion

Systemic
- ↑ Blood pressure
- Diabetes mellitus
- Hyperlipidaemia
- Hyperviscosity syndromes
- Hypercoaguable disorders

Aims

1 Identify the clinical features of central and branch retinal vein occlusion (CRVO and BRVO).
2 Management of CRVO.
3 Management of BRVO.

Skills to obtain

Identify retinal vein occlusion with an ophthalmoscope.

Retinal vein occlusion

Common cause of painless loss of vision—the condition can occur at any age, with 85% of patients aged >50 years. Classified into central (CRVO) and branch (BRVO), depending on the site of the obstruction. The vein is occluded with thrombus, which represents a secondary event following:

- changes to the vascular endothelium;
- external pressure from an overlying arteriole that shares a common adventitial sheath (BRVO);
- increased thrombotic tendency.

Pathology

Exact aetiology is unknown. The resulting venous occlusion causes:

- Increased intravascular pressure:
  —intraretinal haemorrhage;
  —retinal oedema;
  —altered vascular permeability.
- Stagnation of flow:
  —capillary non-perfusion;
  —retinal ischaemia leading to the growth to new vessels at the optic disc, retina or iris.

Visual prognosis depends on the type of occlusion, the severity of the initial insult and the ocular sequelae. Visual loss is worse in CRVO than BRVO. Some small BRVO are asymptomatic, especially if it affects only one quadrant nasal to the disc (i.e. away from the macula)—only a slightly enlarged blind spot is found.

Visual loss may follow:

- **Ischaemic**—vein occlusion affecting the fovea. New vessels give rise to **vitreous haemorrhage** or **neovascular glaucoma**.
- **Exudation**—blood–retinal barrier breakdown causes **macular oedema** and **retinal exudate**.

Central retinal vein occlusion

The CRV deep in the optic cup is occluded, affecting drainage from all four retinal quadrants, resulting in usually unilateral painless visual loss.

Signs

- Afferent pupillary defect common.
- Dilated retinal examination demonstrates:
  —retinal haemorrhages in all four quadrants;
  —optic disc swelling;
  —venous dilation and tortuosity ±cotton wool spots.

Ischaemic CRVO

Up to 33% of cases are ischaemic, associated with new vessel formation on the iris (rubeosis iridis) or disc, a risk of neovascular glaucoma, and vitreous haemorrhage, and blindness. Requires laser treatment.

Signs:

- Deep retinal haemorrhages.
- More than 10 cotton wool spots.
- Large areas of capillary non-perfusion (detected with FFA).

Non-ischaemic CRVO

- Mild fundus changes.
- No afferent papillary defect.
- Visual loss not as profound as in ischaemic CRVO.
- May not require laser treatment.

Branch retinal vein occlusion

Occur at arterovenous crossings and are 3 times more common than CRVOs.

Presents as with CRVO if extensive, or incidental finding. Retinal haemorrhages and cotton wool spots are confined to one area. Chronic retinal changes: exudate, macular oedema and collateral vessels. New vessels arise from the retina rather than the iris, therefore these patients may get a vitreous haemorrhage but not neovascular glaucoma.

Management

In both CRVO and BRVO it is important to detect and treat any underlying systemic disease in order to prevent the recurrence of the venous occlusion.

- **Ophthalmic management**:
  —Check intraocular pressure (IOP) as may cause CRVO.
  —Screen for presence of new vessels (over 2 years).
- **Medical management**:
  —Check FBC, ESR, U&E, lipid profile, blood sugar, plasma proteins and blood pressure.
  —Medical treatment of cardiovascular risk factors.
  —Aspirin.

Treatment

CRVO

- Look for iris neovascularization in ischaemic CRVO—typically occurs at 3 months ('100 day glaucoma').
- Reduce IOP if over 22 mmHg.
- Laser PRP is applied in the presence of new vessels.
- Cyclodiode if advanced and glaucoma.

BRVO

- Follow up BRVO every 4–6 weeks for 6 months. If it worsens and looks ischaemic, use PRP.

Hypertension and the eye

Looking at the retina you are looking at blood vessels in the body, which gives some idea of vascular damage. Severe vascular damage in the general population is uncommon and is seen in special groups, for instance patients with renal failure.

Systemic hypertension	Accelerated hypertension (*rare!*)
Early changes: silver wiring AV nipping Later changes: flame haemorrhages papilloedema	Marked systemic changes plus lots of retinal flame haemorrhages, star exudates at macula, papilloedema, BRVO or CRVO

KEY POINTS

- The CRV drains the entire retina and prelaminar optic nerve head.
- Ischaemic-type CRVO may develop neovascular glaucoma.
- Some BRVOs are asymptomatic, but indicate systemic disease.

45 Retinal artery obstruction

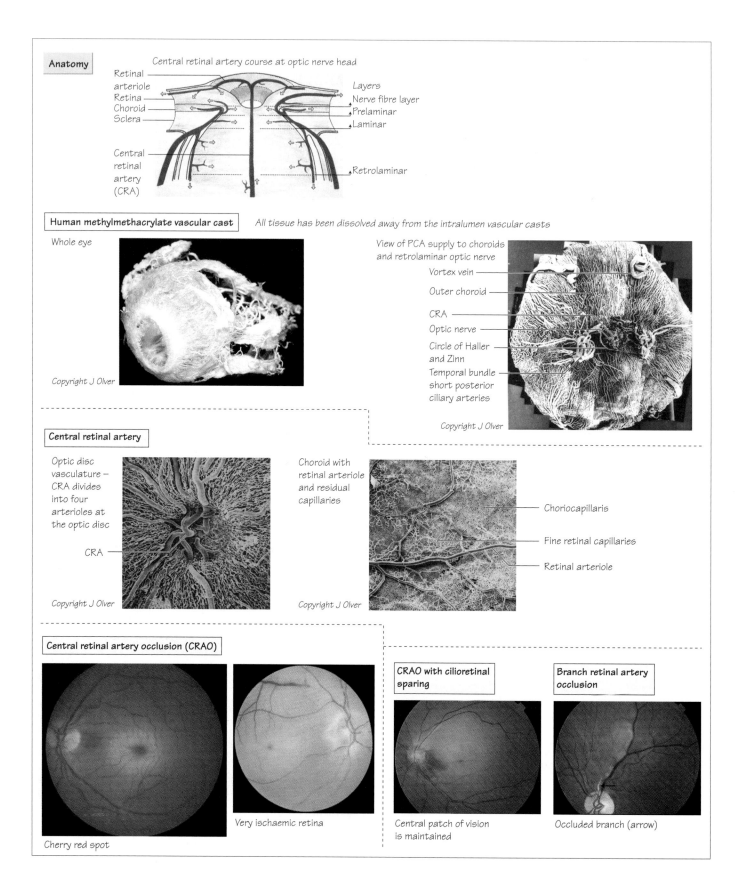

Anatomy

Central retinal artery course at optic nerve head

Retinal arteriole
Retina
Choroid
Sclera

Central retinal artery (CRA)

Layers
Nerve fibre layer
Prelaminar
Laminar
Retrolaminar

Human methylmethacrylate vascular cast — *All tissue has been dissolved away from the intralumen vascular casts*

Whole eye

Copyright J Olver

View of PCA supply to choroids and retrolaminar optic nerve

Vortex vein
Outer choroid
CRA
Optic nerve
Circle of Haller and Zinn
Temporal bundle short posterior ciliary arteries

Copyright J Olver

Central retinal artery

Optic disc vasculature – CRA divides into four arterioles at the optic disc

CRA

Copyright J Olver

Choroid with retinal arteriole and residual capillaries

Choriocapillaris
Fine retinal capillaries
Retinal arteriole

Copyright J Olver

Central retinal artery occlusion (CRAO)

Cherry red spot

Very ischaemic retina

CRAO with cilioretinal sparing

Central patch of vision is maintained

Branch retinal artery occlusion

Occluded branch (arrow)

Aims

1 Understand the vascular anatomy of the retina and optic nerve head.
2 Identify the clinical features of a central retinal artery occlusion (CRAO).
3 Be able to manage a patient with CRAO.

Anatomy

The eye has a rich blood supply from the ophthalmic artery via the central retinal artery (CRA) and the posterior ciliary arteries (PCAs). The CRA supplies the superficial nerve fibre layer and inner two-thirds of the retina. The PCAs supply the rest of the anterior optic nerve and uvea (iris, ciliary body and choroid), and hence the deep retinal layers. The anatomy is known from vascular casts (*in vitro*) and fluorescein angiography.

In vascular casts of the eye the cadaver ophthalmic artery has been injected with a plastic and the tissue has been dissolved away leaving only the vessel lumen—the cast.

The CRA is an end artery of the ophthalmic artery, which supplies the inner two-thirds of the retina. The choriocapillaris supplies the outer retina.

> **WARNING**
> CRA obstruction causes ischaemia of the inner retinal layers resulting in oedema of the nerve fibre layer (NFL).
> **Urgent**: If bloodflow is not restored within 100 min, irreversible damage occurs at its narrowest point, which is the lamina cribrosa. A blockage more distally gives rise to a branch artery occlusion.

Pathology

Arterial occlusion results from	Inner retinal ischaemia causes	Retinal infarction gives rise to
• Circulating embolus (e.g. heart, carotids) • Local atheroma • Arteritis (e.g. giant cell arteritis) • Miscellaneous (e.g. migraine, syphilis, herpes zoster)	• Intracellular oedema— the retina appears white which masks the choroidal circulation, except at the macula 'cherry red spot'	• Loss of NFL • Pale optic disc

Cilioretinal artery

NB, 15–20% of individuals have a supplementary arterial supply to the macula via a cilioretinal artery derived from the posterior ciliary circulation at the disc. In the event of a CRAO, the macula would remain perfused in these patients with some preservation of vision.

Diagnosis and management

Symptoms

• Painless loss of vision (NB, non-ocular pain may occur such as temporal or scalp tenderness in giant cell arteritis (GCA)).
• Profound drop in visual acuity (unless cilioretinal artery sparing).
• Afferent papillary defect.

Signs

Perform a dilated fundal examination to detect:
• Cherry red spot at macula.
• Embolus occasionally visible at optic disc.
• Attenuation of arterioles.
• Retinal pallor.
• Mild disc swelling.

Treatment

The aim is to re-establish circulation within the CRA. This is attempted by:
• Lowering the intraocular pressure (IOP) using:
 —acetazolamide 500 mg i.v.;
 —ocular massage;
 —anterior chamber paracentesis (1 ml aqueous withdrawn).
• Vasodilation: rebreathe into a paper bag (carbon dioxide increases).
• Start cholesterol lowering statins, e.g. Simvastatin, Atorvastatin.
• Start antiplatelets, e.g. aspirin 300 mg stat then 75 mg daily or clopidogrel 75 mg daily, within 48 hrs.

> **WARNING**
> It is *essential* to check the erythrocyte sedimentation rate (ESR) and CRP to investigate for an inflammatory cause for CRAO, since GCA is often a bilateral condition with catastrophic visual loss if not treated appropriately.

Outcome

Visual recovery is dependent on the interval between onset and presentation. There has not been a clinical trial comparing treatment versus no treatment—but it is believed that 66% of patients have vision <6/60 following CRAO.

Other investigations

Examine for carotid bruits, heart murmurs and irregular pulse (atrial fibrillation is a cause—needs anticoagulation). Arrange carotid Doppler studies, 24 h Holter monitor and echocardiogram. Follow-up by a physician.

KEY POINTS

• The CRA supplies the inner two-thirds of the retina.
• Do an ESR in all cases of CRAO to exclude GCA.
• A cilioretinal artery is present in 15–20% of individuals, which affords some protection from severe visual loss.

- AIDS (acquired immune deficiency syndrome) is caused by infection with HIV (human immunodeficiency virus). It was first described in 1981 in the USA and is now a global pandemic
- The number of reported cases underestimates the true extent of this infection with over 75% of cases occurring in sub-Saharan Africa, where the major mode of transmission is heterosexual sex
- The incidence of heterosexual transmission is increasing in the USA, Europe and Australia whereas intravenous drug users (IVDU) and homosexual transmission is plateauing
- HIV infects cells by attachment to the CD4 antigen complex found on many cells (CD4 cells, B-lymphocytes, macrophages, cells in CNS)

Eyelids

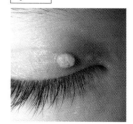

Molluscum contagiosum on eyelid (usually multiple in HIV)

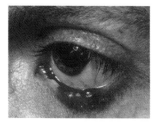

Kaposi sarcoma lower eyelid

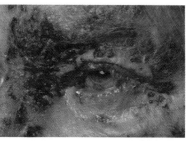

Herpes zoster ophthalmicus (5i) plus maxillary branch involvement (5ii)

Intraocular inflammation

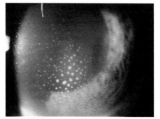

Anterior uveitis with granulomatous keratoprecipitates

Retinal ischaemia

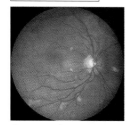

Cotton wool spots

Retinal/choroidal infections

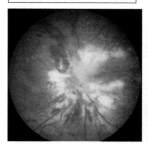
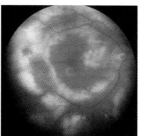

Cytomegalovirus (CMV) papillitis and chorioretinitis

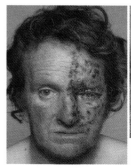

Varicella zoster virus retinitis (VZVR)

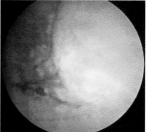

Toxoplasmosis retinochoroiditis

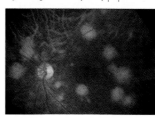

Pneumocystis carinii pneumonia (PCP) choroiditis

Visual prognosis:
VZVR, CMV, toxoplasmosis retinochoroiditis and candida endophthalmitis may cause severe visual loss.
PCP and cryptococcal retinitis is treatable

WARNING

Varicella zoster virus retinitis (VZVR) – may blind patients
- Acute retinal necrosis (ARN) and progressive outer retinal necrosis (PORN) when immunocompetent and immunosuppressed
- PORN: bilateral multifocal retinitis with opacification in the outer retina and rapid progression. Minimal or no vitritis. Very poor prognosis with standard therapies, leading to blindness in most cases

HIV modes of transmission

- Sexual transmission (homosexual and heterosexual)
- Parenteral transmission with blood and blood products: semen from artificial insemination and organ transplantation
- Occupational risk: small risk for healthcare workers of 0.3% after a single percutaneous exposure to HIV-infected blood. Infection risk also from blood contamination of mucous membranes, non-intact skin and conjunctiva
- Perinatal transmission: accounts for 80–90% of all paediatric HIV infections. Congenital HIV infection may occur transplacentally or intrapartum. The majority of infection occurs during birth or from breastfeeding
- Other routes: no evidence of HIV transmission from tears, sweat, urine or other body fluids
- NB. 30–50% of the non-HIV population will have serological evidence of previous toxoplasmosis

Aims

1 Modes of transmission of HIV (no evidence via tears).
2 Lid, anterior segment, orbit, retinal and neuro-ophthalmic manifestations.
3 Causes of permanent visual loss in HIV.

Ophthalmologic disorders in HIV

Ophthalmic problems in AIDS are common and range from mild conjunctivitis to sight-threatening retinitis. Any ocular or orbital tissue may be involved. The commonest and most important opportunistic infection is **cytomegalovirus retinitis** (CMVR).

Lids/conjunctiva

- Trichomegaly—long eyelashes.
- Molluscum contagiosum on eyelids.
- HIV-related conjunctivitis.
- HIV conjunctival microvasculopathy—dilated, corkscrew-like, tortuous vessels seen on slit lamp examination.
- Kaposi's sarcoma—flat or raised (if present >4/12) violaceous vascular lesion, surrounded by tortuous and dilated vessels. Common in conjunctival fornix. Treated by excision, chemotherapy or radiotherapy.
- Conjunctival granulomas due to cryptococcal infection, tuberculosis and other mycotic infections.
- Squamous cell carcinoma (see Chapter 24). Associated with human papillomavirus infection. Aggressive tumour found on the lid or conjunctiva.
- Herpes zoster opthalmicus (HZO) often affects the VIIth nerve too.

Cornea/anterior uveitis

- Anterior uveitis from drug toxicity (rifabutin, cidofovir).
- Herpes simplex keratitis.
- HZO keratitis.
- Microsporidia: a protozoal infection causing coarse, superficial, punctate keratitis with minimal conjunctival reaction.

Orbital disease

- Periorbital B cell lymphoma.
- *Aspergillus* mass.
- Burkitt's lymphoma.
- Kaposi's sarcoma.

Retinal disease

HIV retinopathy

- Cotton wool spots.
- Retinal haemorrhages.
- Microaneurysms.
- Ischaemic maculopathy.
- Immune recovery uveitis (IRU). Occurs in eye with quiescent CMVR in patients responding to HAART, defined as vitritis of ≥1+ *or* trace of cells + epiretinal membrane *or* cystoid macular oedema.

Retinal infections

Cytomegalovirus retinitis (CMVR)
Haemorrhagic or non-haemorrhagic, frosted-branch angiitis or mimic central retinal vein occlusion.

Epstein–Barr virus (EBV) retinitis
Multifocal choroidal inflammation; typically prodromal malaise. EBV DNA is present in normal ocular tissue hence its presence in vitreous biopsy is not conclusive evidence of EBV uveitis.

Toxoplasmosis retinochoroiditis (*Toxoplasma gondii*)
- White or yellow patch of focal retinal necrosis. In HIV lesions tend to be larger; bilateral disease in 18–38%; unusual forms occur (solitary, multifocal or miliary), often there is no pre-existing scar; minimal vitritis; prolonged therapy is required.

Syphilitic retinitis
Myriad presentations—vitritis, multifocal choroiditis, retinal vasculitis, neuroretinitis, optic atrophy or oedema, exudative retinal detachment, choroidal effusion, pigmentary retinopathy, and venous and arterial occlusions.

Cryptococcal choroiditis (*Cryptococcus neoformans*)
Variably-sized deep choroidal infiltrates; may be asymptomatic.

Pneumocystis carinii choroiditis
Superficial yellow-white choroidal lesions.

Mycobacterium tuberculosis choroiditis
Single large granuloma or multifocal; ±retinal vasculitis; frequently bilateral; choroidal neovascularization may develop at sites of healed spots.

Mycobacterium avium-intracellulare choroiditis
Similar to multifocal choroiditis seen in cryptococcal and *Pneumocystis carinii* pneumonia (PCP) infection.

Candida endophthalmitis (*Candida albicans*)
Small, whitish, multifocal, circumscribed chorioretinal infiltrates; retinal haems; dense vitritis and 'fluff balls' (vitreous abscesses) progress to endophthalmitis; often IVDU.

Aspergillus endophthalmitis
Dense vitritis and vitreoretinal abscesses (similar to *Candida* infection).

Ocular histoplasmosis infection (*Histoplasma capsulatum*)
Endophthalmitis (iritis, vitritis, yellow iris infiltrates, multiple creamy foci of retinochoroiditis + pulmonary or disseminated infection) or solitary chorioretinal granuloma (±vitritis).

Primary intraocular B cell lymphoma
Typically high grade; significant vitritis ± iritis; peripapillary infiltrates; disc swelling; yellow-white sub-RPE lesions; vascular sheathing; and vein or artery occlusion.

Neuro-ophthalmic disorders in HIV

- Optic disc swelling secondary to cryptococcal meningitis.
- Papilloedema secondary to progressive multifocal leucoencephalopathy (PML), cerebral infarction, intracranial toxoplasmosis or lymphoma.
- Optic atrophy secondary to retinal disease.
- Visual field defects secondary to space-occupying lesions.
- Cranial nerve palsies secondary to intracranial SOL or infection.
- Unilateral facial palsy may be secondary to aseptic meningitis.

KEY POINTS

- No evidence that HIV is transmitted from tears.
- HZO or multiple molluscum contagiosum in a young adult may indicate HIV.
- Increased orbital B cell lymphoma in HIV.

47 Pupil abnormalities

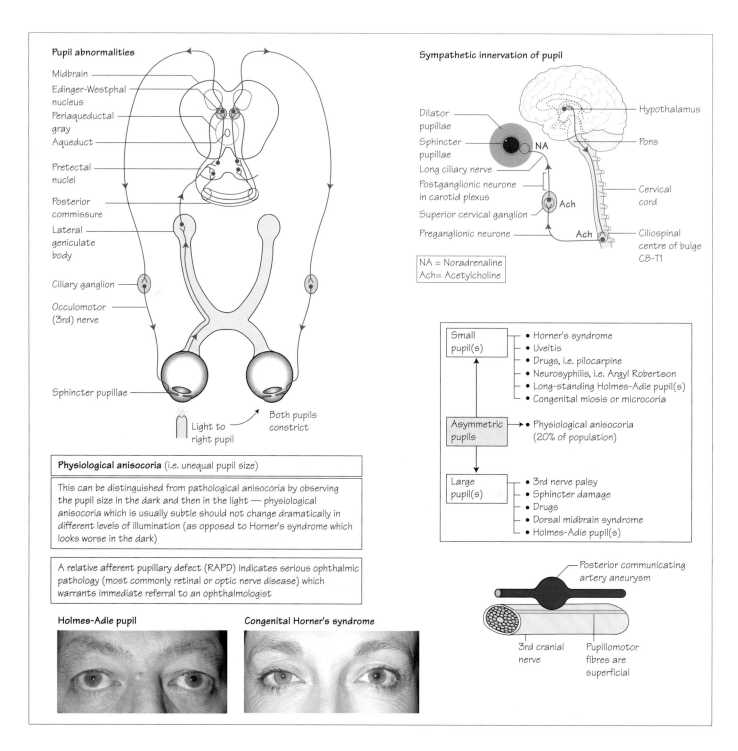

Pupil abnormalities

- Midbrain
- Edinger-Westphal nucleus
- Periaqueductal gray
- Aqueduct
- Pretectal nuclei
- Posterior commissure
- Lateral geniculate body
- Ciliary ganglion
- Occulomotor (3rd) nerve
- Sphincter pupillae

Light to right pupil

Both pupils constrict

Sympathetic innervation of pupil

- Dilator pupillae
- Sphincter pupillae
- Long ciliary nerve
- Postganglionic neurone in carotid plexus
- Superior cervical ganglion
- Preganglionic neurone
- Hypothalamus
- Pons
- Cervical cord
- Ciliospinal centre of bulge C8-T1

NA = Noradrenaline
Ach = Acetylcholine

Physiological anisocoria (i.e. unequal pupil size)

This can be distinguished from pathological anisocoria by observing the pupil size in the dark and then in the light — physiological anisocoria which is usually subtle should not change dramatically in different levels of illumination (as opposed to Horner's syndrome which looks worse in the dark)

A relative afferent pupillary defect (RAPD) indicates serious ophthalmic pathology (most commonly retinal or optic nerve disease) which warrants immediate referral to an ophthalmologist

Holmes-Adie pupil

Congenital Horner's syndrome

Small pupil(s)
- Horner's syndrome
- Uveitis
- Drugs, i.e. pilocarpine
- Neurosyphilis, i.e. Argyl Robertson
- Long-standing Holmes-Adie pupil(s)
- Congenital miosis or microcoria

Asymmetric pupils
- Physiological anisocoria (20% of population)

Large pupil(s)
- 3rd nerve palsy
- Sphincter damage
- Drugs
- Dorsal midbrain syndrome
- Holmes-Adie pupil(s)

- Posterior communicating artery aneurysm
- 3rd cranial nerve
- Pupillomotor fibres are superficial

Aims
1 Understand how to assess a patient with abnormal pupils.
2 Understand the causes of pupil abnormalities.
3 Understand the neuroanatomy of pupillary light reflexes.

Pupil examination
When examining pupils you need to check for:
- Symmetry.
- Size.
- Shape.
- Light response.
- Near response.

Afferent pupil defect (APD) / relative afferent pupillary defect (RAPD)
- An APD results from damage to the visual pathway anywhere

from the retinal ganglion cell layer to the lateral geniculate body, thus causing a reduction in the input (afferent) signal reaching the brainstem when a light is directed at the affected eye. Hence there is a similarly reduced output (efferent) signal reaching the pupil, which consequently constricts to a lesser extent than if it had received a full signal.

• Because of the consensual light reflex, the unaffected pupil will also constrict to an equally lesser extent when the light is directed towards the damaged side.

• Hence, if a light is directed at the better eye both pupils will constrict fully and equally. If it is the immediately swung over ('swinging flash light test') and directed at the affected eye (e.g. an eye with an optic nerve lesion) both pupils will appear to dilate—RAPD. In fact what has happened here is that both pupils are constricting but to a lesser degree than when the light was directed at the normal eye, hence they only appear to dilate. When the light is swung back to the better eye the pupils will constrict.

Fixed dilated pupil

• If a pupil is dilated and doesn't react to light or accommodation, it is important to examine eye movements and levator function in order to exclude a **third nerve palsy**. NB, a unilateral enlarged pupil caused by uncal herniation is a neurosurgical emergency.

• Because of the superficial location of the pupillomotor fibres (see figure), a partial third nerve palsy can occur where only the pupil is involved. In such cases a **tumour** or **posterior communicating artery aneurysm** must be excluded.

• A fixed dilated pupil can result from inadvertent or accidental contamination of the eye with **cycloplegic agents** such as atropine or cyclopentolate, hence the importance of a detailed history.

• Previous **trauma** or **surgery** where there has been extensive damage to the sphincter pupillae can result in a fixed dilated pupil.

• A fixed semidilated pupil in the presence of a hazy cornea, red eye and pain is seen in **acute angle-closure glaucoma**.

Small pupil (miosis)

• A small pupil in association with a very small amount of ptosis (no more than 2 mm—due to paralysis of Müller's muscle) is known as **Horner's syndrome**. This results from a lesion of the sympathetic chain anywhere from the hypothalmus to the eye.

• On dimming the lights the anisocoria will become more obvious as the affected pupil doesn't dilate in the dark as well as its counterpart.

• There may be other associated features such as elevation of the lower lid, which together with the ptosis gives the appearance of enophthalmos, reduced sweating on the ipsilateral side of the face and occasionally conjunctival hyperaemia.

• Horner's syndrome can be confirmed by putting 4% cocaine drops into each eye and observing the pupils 40 min later. The normal pupil will dilate, the Horner's pupil will not.

• Causes of Horner's syndrome include Pancoast's tumour of the lung, thoracic aortic aneurysm, trauma, carotid artery dissection (usually accompanied by neck pain) and CNS disease. All patients should be investigated appropriately.

• In **congenital Horner's syndrome** the iris on the affected side is a different colour—iris heterochromia.

• Contamination of the eye with **pilocarpine** causes miosis.

• Uveitis that has resulted in **posterior synechiae** can result in a small pupil.

• Rarely, **congenital microcoria** can occur.

Light–near dissociation

In some cases the pupil(s) will accommodate but not react to light. This dissociation of the light and near reflex can occur in various syndromes.

• **Dorsal midbrain** or **Parinaud's syndrome**. This may be due to a lesion (e.g. pinealoma, cranipharyngioma) compressing the pupillary light reflex fibres. The pupils may be large and eccentric. Associated features include absence of upgaze, upper lid retraction and convergence retraction nystagmus, characterized by rapid convergence movements and retraction of both eyes on attempted upgaze.

• **Neurosyphilis** or **Argyll Robertson pupils**. These pupils are small and irregular, do not react to light but react briskly to near stimuli.

• **Holmes–Adie pupil**. This is thought to result from a viral infection; the affected pupil is initially large and eventually may become miosed. There is no reaction to light, the near reflex is intact but delayed and tonic (the patient should be asked to focus on a near target for at least 1 min before the pupils begin to constrict, and when the patient is then asked to relax his accommodation the pupils are slow to dilate again). These patients may also have absent tendon reflexes. Both pupils may eventually become involved.

• Patients with **Myotonic dystrophy** may have light–near dissociation.

• Patients with **diabetes** may develop a **pupil neuropathy** resulting in light–near dissociation.

KEY POINTS
• Fixed dilated pupil—'surgical third' must be outruled.
• Unilateral miosis—Horner's syndrome must be outruled.
• RAPD—indicates optic nerve or retinal disease.

Features of optic atrophy and papilloedema

Reduced visual acuity

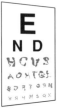
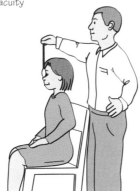
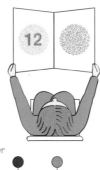

Reduced
visual
acuity

Reduced colour vision

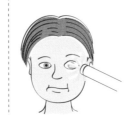

or

Red desaturation

Relative afferent
pupillary defect

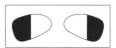
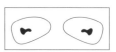

Visual field loss

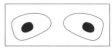

Enlarged blind spot in papilloedema

Centrocaecal scotoma in Lebers optic
atrophy or vitamin B12 deficiency

Bitemporal hemianopia in optic
atrophy 2°E pituitary tumour

Swollen discs

Multiple sclerosis (MS)

Pale

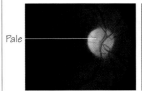

Right unilateral optic
atrophy in MS

Left disc normal

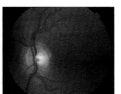
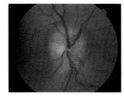

Acute right papillitis
(swollen disc) in MS
optic neuritis

Left nerve is normal

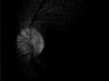

Right optic
nerve higher
signal than
left

Coronal MRI scan showing
demyelination and high
signal in right optic nerve

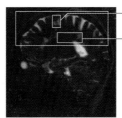

— Demyelinating
plaque
— Dawson's fingers

Sagittal MRI scan showing
demyelination involving the
corpus callosum

Benign intracranial hypertension (BIH)

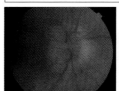
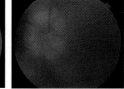

Bilateral chronic papilloedema secondary to BIH

Leber's Hereditary Optic Neuropathy (LHON)

- A hereditary optic neuropathy affecting young males 20–30 years
- Mitochondrial inheritance (i.e. passed via mitochondrial DNA) passed through female side of the family in most cases
- Often smokers
- Presents with
  - Subacute painless loss of central vision in one or both eyes
  - Second eye involved within weeks–months
  - Centrocaecal scotoma
  - Typical circumpapillary telangiectatic microangiopathy

The primary mutation has prognostic implications:

11778 - 2–17% recovery
3460 - 15–30% recovery
14484 - 37–50% recovery

- Treatment : none, advise to stop smoking

Leber's Hereditary Optic Neuropathy – bilateral involvement

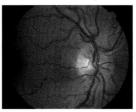
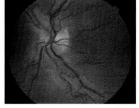

Blurred nasal disc margins and pre-capillary telangiectasis

Typically discs swollen in the acute phase

Aims
Know the causes of optic atrophy (pale disc) and swollen discs.

Optic atrophy/neuropathy
Clinical features
- VA is reduced, but can be normal, depending on the degree of optic atrophy.
- In those patients with subtle optic atrophy and apparently normal visual acuity, colour vision may be reduced and a visual field defect present. Formal perimetry is essential, but confrontational fields using a red target can be most informative.
- Relative afferent pupillary defect.
- Disc pallor. In severe optic atrophy the entire disc may be pale, in many cases only part of the disc (e.g. the temporal part) will be affected and subtle disc pallor will be missed if both discs are not compared.

Aetiology
- **Hereditary:**
  —Autosomal dominant optic atrophy: visual acuity may be minimally reduced. Affected family members may vary considerably in abnormalities.
  —Autosomal recessive optic atrophy: poor visual acuity.
  —Leber's hereditary optic atrophy (LHON), (see figure).
- **Retinal dystrophy:**
  —Cone dystrophy: very poor acuity, markedly reduced colour vision, photophobia, central scotoma, nystagmus, typical ERG.
  —Retinitis pigmentosa: typical retinal appearance, constricted visual fields and characteristic electroretinogram (ERG).
- **Vascular:** central retinal artery occlusion (history of angina or peripheral vascular disease and sudden profound loss of vision, typical fundal appearance in acute phase—cherry red spot, arteriolar attenuation).
- **Nutritional/toxic:** vitamin B_{12} deficiency (gradual bilateral visual loss associated with pins and needles in hands and feet, poor diet, reduced colour vision, centrocaecal scotoma), tobacco–alcohol amblyopia or drugs (e.g. ethambutol, chloramphenicol).
- **Inflammatory:** sarcoidosis, polyarteritis nodosa, contiguous sinus disease—more commonly present with disc swelling.
- **Demyelination** (may have past history of typical attacks of optic neuritis, and may have other neurological symptoms). It is a common cause.
- **Compressive:** optic nerve glioma or meningioma, orbital tumour or intracranial tumour.

Investigations
- Formal visual field testing.
- Visual evoked response/potential (VER/VEP).
- ERG.
- Relevant blood tests depending on clinical history (e.g. vitamin B_{12} and folate levels in a patient who is a vegan and has bilateral optic atrophy with glove and stocking paraesthesia).
- Neuroimaging: MRI optic nerves and brain

Disc swelling
Unilateral disc swelling
Clinical features
- Visual acuity may be normal or reduced.
- Reduced colour vision.
- Visual field defect: enlarged blind spot if there is significant swelling; altitudinal defect if disc swelling is secondary to ischaemic optic neuropathy.
- Blurred disc margin ± splinter haemorrhages (see figure).

Aetiology
- Vascular: e.g. AION, CRV or diabetic papillopathy.
- Inflammatory: 'papillitis', e.g. uveitis, sarcoidosis, viral, systemic lupus erythematosus or paranasal sinus disease.
- Demyelination: multiple sclerosis—disc swelling may become bilateral. Disc(s) swollen or normal in acute phase, and eventually become pale after recurrent attacks.
- Hereditary: LHON—may become bilateral.
- Infiltrative: e.g. lymphoma.
- Infective: e.g. toxoplasmosis, herpes or Lyme's disease.

Investigations
- Visual field analysis.
- Full blood count (FBC), blood glucose, ESR, CRP, coagulation screen, infective screen (e.g. toxoplasmosis and *Borelia* titres), autoantibody screen.
- Blood sent for analysis for Leber's mutation if suspected.
- Neuroimaging if demyelination or a compressive lesion is suspected. MRI of the brain and optic nerves should be requested.
- Lumbar puncture if demyelination, neurosarcoidosis or lymphoma are suspected.

Bilateral disc swelling/papilloedema
Clinical features
- Visual acuity may be normal or severely reduced.
- Patients with papilloedema may complain of episodes of unilateral or bilateral transient visual loss lasting for a few seconds. These are transient visual obscurations (TVOs) and can be precipitated by changes in posture.
- Colour vision is often reduced.
- Enlarged blind spot if the swelling is significant; it will be normal in mild cases.

Aetiology
- Raised intracranial pressure: SOL, hydrocephalus, benign/idiopathic intracranial hypertension (BIH/IIH).
- Malignant hypertension.
- Diabetic papillopathy.
- Infiltrative papilloedema, e.g. lymphoma.
- Toxic, e.g. ethambutol or chloramphenicol uraemia.

Investigations
- Blood pressure.
- Glucose, FBC and differential WCC, U&E, creatinine and ESR.
- Neuroimaging.
- Lumbar puncture if the MRI is normal and BIH is suspected.
- Visual fields (to monitor blind spot).

KEY POINTS
- Rule out malignant hypertension in papilloedema.
- *Urgent* CT brain if headache, nausea, papilloedema, normal BP.
- MRI if demyelination suspected.

49 Cranial nerve palsies and eye movement disorders

Neuroanatomy of the 3rd, 4th, 6th and 7th cranial nerves

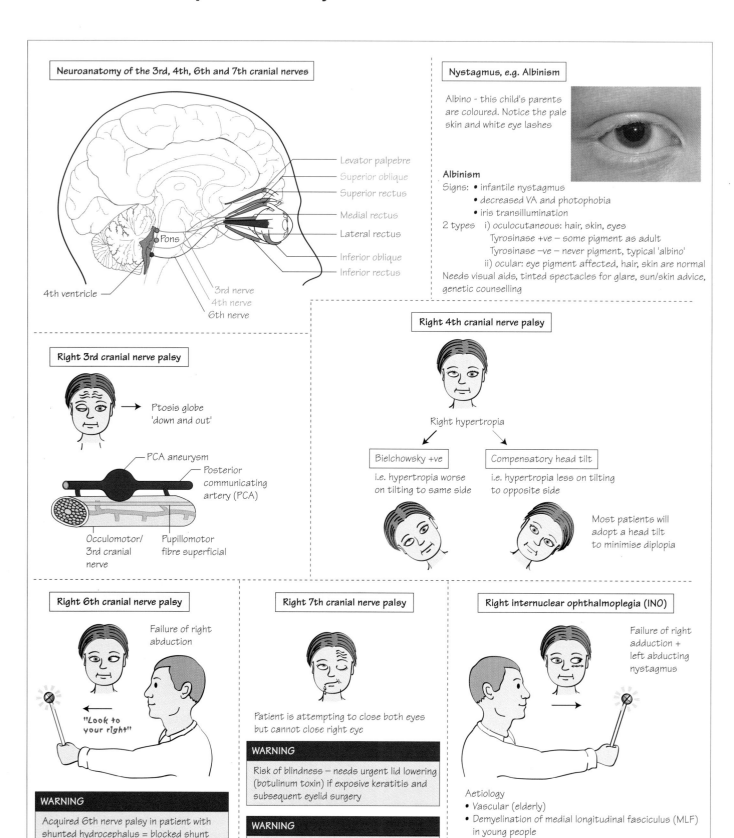

Levator palpebre
Superior oblique
Superior rectus
Medial rectus
Lateral rectus
Inferior oblique
Inferior rectus

4th ventricle
Pons
3rd nerve
4th nerve
6th nerve

Nystagmus, e.g. Albinism

Albino - this child's parents are coloured. Notice the pale skin and white eye lashes

Albinism

Signs: • infantile nystagmus
• decreased VA and photophobia
• iris transillumination

2 types i) oculocutaneous: hair, skin, eyes
Tyrosinase +ve – some pigment as adult
Tyrosinase –ve – never pigment, typical 'albino'
ii) ocular: eye pigment affected, hair, skin are normal

Needs visual aids, tinted spectacles for glare, sun/skin advice, genetic counselling

Right 3rd cranial nerve palsy

Ptosis globe 'down and out'

PCA aneurysm
Posterior communicating artery (PCA)

Occulomotor/ 3rd cranial nerve
Pupillomotor fibre superficial

Right 4th cranial nerve palsy

Right hypertropia

Bielchowsky +ve	Compensatory head tilt
i.e. hypertropia worse on tilting to same side	i.e. hypertropia less on tilting to opposite side

Most patients will adopt a head tilt to minimise diplopia

Right 6th cranial nerve palsy

Failure of right abduction

"Look to your right"

WARNING

Acquired 6th nerve palsy in patient with shunted hydrocephalus = blocked shunt = emergency

Right 7th cranial nerve palsy

Patient is attempting to close both eyes but cannot close right eye

WARNING

Risk of blindness – needs urgent lid lowering (botulinum toxin) if expsove keratitis and subsequent eyelid surgery

WARNING

Management, investigate, surgery

Right internuclear ophthalmoplegia (INO)

Failure of right adduction + left abducting nystagmus

Aetiology
• Vascular (elderly)
• Demyelination of medial longitudinal fasciculus (MLF) in young people
• Needs MRI brainstem

Aim

- Describe clinical features of IIIrd, IVth, VIth and VIIth cranial nerve palsies, internuclear ophthalmoplegia (INO), gaze palsies and nystagmus.

Third nerve palsy

Symptoms
- Double vision—horizontal and/or vertical.
- Droopy lid.
- Enlarged pupil.
- Headache. NB, painful third with pupil involvement—exclude posterior communicating artery aneurysm as soon as possible.

Signs
- Ptosis.
- Exotropia and hypotropia (globe appears down and out).
- Fixed dilated pupil.
- Limitation of elevation, depression, and adduction.
May present with any of these or combination.

Aetiology
- Ischaemic/vascular (usually pupil sparing due to anatomy of the pupillomotor fibres, and referred to as a 'medical third'): diabetes mellitus (DM), hypertension, vasculitis or migraine.
- Compressive lesion (pupil nearly always involved, and referred to as a 'surgical third'): posterior communicating artery aneurysm, tumour.
- Trauma.
- Congenital third.

Fourth nerve palsy

Symptoms
Double vision—vertical.

Signs
- Head tilt opposite to the side of the lesion.
- Hypertropia on the affected side.
- Limitation of eye movement down and to the right if left fourth nerve palsy, and visa versa.
- Positive Bielchowsky's sign, i.e. the hypertropia on the affected side gets worse on tilting the head to the same side.

Aetiology
- Trauma is the most common cause of IVth nerve palsy as has the longest intracranial course, is very slender and runs under the tentorial edge. Trauma may result in bilateral fourths.
- Ischaemic/vascular: DM, hypertension or vasculitis.
- Compressive lesion, e.g. intracranial tumour.
- Congenital.

Fifth nerve palsy

Corneal anaesthesia.

Sixth nerve palsy

Symptoms
Double vision—horizontal.

Signs
- Esotropia, worse for distance.
- Limitation of abduction of the affected eye.

Aetiology
- Vascular/ischaemic: DM, hypertension, or vasculitis.
- Invading intracranial or nasopharyngeal tumour.
- Trauma, e.g. fractured skull base.

Seventh nerve palsy

Symptoms
- Inability to close eyelid (lagophthalmos) and facial weakness.

- Watery eye (due to weakness of orbicularis oculi).
- Sore red eye (due to corneal exposure).
- Blurred vision secondary to exposure keratitis.
- Drooling.

Signs
- Ipsilateral facial muscle weakness, involving the frontalis in lower motor neurone lesions. The frontalis is spared in upper motor neurone lesions.
- Lower lid ectropion secondary to orbicularis oculi weakness.
- Corneal exposure may vary from superficial punctate erosions to corneal abrasion, and must be treated urgently to prevent abscess formation and endophthalmitis.

> **WARNING**
> May have Vth nerve palsy and corneal anaesthesia.

Aetiology
- Viral/idiopahtic, e.g. Bell's palsy (usually improves spontaneously) or Ramsay–Hunt syndrome (herpes simplex infection).
- Compressive lesion: intracranial tumour, e.g. acoustic neuroma (may have associated Vth, VIth and VIIIth nerve palsy) or parotid tumour.
- Vascular/ischaemic: DM, hypertension or vasculitis.
- Inflammation, e.g. sarcoidosis.

Internuclear ophthalmoplegia

Symptoms
- Horizontal diplopia.
- Inability to coordinate eye movements.

Signs
- Failure to adduct the ipsilateral eye.
- Abducting nystagmus of the contralateral eye.

Gaze palsies

Symptoms
- Usually asymptomatic.
- May be unable to move eyes together to one side.

Signs
- Failure to move both eyes to one side.
- Both eyes may be deviated to one side.

Aetiology
Lesion affecting the supranuclear (i.e. the neural pathways superior to the IIIrd, IVth and VIth nerve nuclei) pathways in the cerebral cortex or brainstem, e.g. stroke, demyelination or SOL.

Nystagmus

This is involuntary rhythmic to-and-fro oscillation of the eyes.

Symptoms
- Congenital nystagmus is asymptomatic.
- Acquired nystagmus may cause oscillopsia, a sensation of rapid movement or oscillation of the visual environment. Patients describe it as though looking at an old black and white film where everything flickers or wobbles; others notice only blurred vision, especially if gaze-evoked nystagmus.

> **WARNING**
> Refer any patient with nystagmus for prompt assessment by a neuro-ophthalmologist to exclude intracranial SOL.

KEY POINTS
- Painful third—posterior communicating artery aneurysm.
- Traumatic sixth—basal skull fracture.
- Internuclear ophthalmoplegia—demyelination.

A detailed knowledge of the neuroanatomy of the visual pathway can help the clinician to localize lesions from the field defect found

Left temporal field
Left nasal field
Right nasal field
Right temporal field

Nasal retina

Temporal retina

Optic nerve

Von Willbrand's knee

Optic tract

Chiasm

Lateral geniculate body

Meyer's loop

Inferior horn of lateral ventricle

Optic radiation

Occipital visual cortex

Left   Right

1 Optic nerve

1a **Superior arcuate scotoma**
e.g. glaucoma

1b **Inferior arcuate scotoma**
e.g. glaucoma

1c **Centrocaecal scotoma**
e.g. B12 deficiency optic neuropathy
Leber's optic neuropathy

1d **Superior altitudinal defect**
e.g. aion or pion

1e **Inferior altitudinal defect**
e.g. aion or pion

2 Junction optic nerve with chiasm

Junctional scotoma
e.g. pit tumour, suprasellar meningioma,
craniopharyngioma, supraclinoid aneurysm

3 Chiasm

Bitemporal hemianopia
i.e. pit tumour, chiasmal glioma,
meningioma, sarcoidosis, MS, abscess

4 Optic tract

Incongruous left homonymous hemianopia
optic tract lesion, i.e. glioma, MS,
metastasis

5 Meyer's loop

Left superior quadrantinopia
i.e. temporal lobe lesion ('pie in the sky')

6 Parietal lobe fibres

Left homonymous hemianopia
denser below, i.e. parietal lobe lesion
(mnemiopic LP = **l**ower **p**arietal)

7 Posterior optic radiation

Congruous left hemianopia

8 Deep occipital cortex

Left homonymous hemianopia with macular sparing, e.g. SOL, MS, trauma, vasculitis

9 Macular fibres at occipital cortex

Central scotomatous left hemianopia,
e.g. SOL, MS, trauma, vascular constriction

10 Retina

Grossly constricted fields – retinal
dystrophy, e.g. RP or severe BIH

Aims

1 Understand the neuroanatomy of the various visual field defects.
2 Recognize the causes of different field defects.

Visual field defects

The most common visual field defects encountered in clinical practice include homonymous hemianopia, altitudinal field defect, bitemporal hemianopia, grossly constricted fields, and enlarged blind spots.

Note obvious clues that will help you, e.g. a hemiparesis—this patient is most likely to have an ipsilateral hemianopia as the result of a lesion in the contralateral cortex (see figure).

1 Optic nerve

A unilateral optic nerve lesion can result in various unilateral field defects depending on the nature of the lesion. The shape of field defect can give a clue to the diagnosis. For example:

• Glaucomatous cupping can result in an **arcuate scotoma** of the superior (1a on figure) or inferior field (1b).
• Vitamin B_{12} deficiency can result in a **centrocaecal scotoma** (1c on figure).
• Anterior ischaemic optic neuropathy (a swollen disc can be seen in the acute phase) and posterior ischaemic optic neuropathy (the disc will look normal in the acute phase) can result in an **altitudinal field defect**. This can be superior (1d on figure) or inferior (1e), depending on which vessels are involved.
• Complete severing of the optic nerve (e.g. as a result of trauma) will cause **complete ipsilateral visual field loss**.

2 Junction optic nerve with chiasm

Because of the arrangement of nerve fibres in the optic nerve and chiasm, a lesion pressing on the visual pathway at the junction of the intracranial optic nerve and the chiasm can produce a characteristic field defect (2 on figure), known as a **junctional scotoma**. Such a field defect results because the lesion compresses both fibres from the nasal fibres (serving the temporal visual field) of the ipsilateral optic nerve and the inferonasal fibres (superotemporal field) from the contralateral eye in Willbrand's knee.

3 Chiasm

A lesion pressing on the optic chiasm, such as a pituitary tumour, will result in damage to the nasal fibres from both eyes as they cross the midline, and therefore results in a **bitemporal hemianopia** (3 on figure). Early on, if the lesion is only minimally compressing the chiasm, the field defect will be very subtle, and may only be picked up by using a red target (the individual will have red desaturation in the affected field—this is true for all subtle lesions).

4 Optic tract

A lesion of the optic tract involves the temporal fibres (nasal field) from the ipsilateral eye and the crossed nasal fibres (temporal field) from the contralateral eye. A lesion completely destroying, for example the right optic tract, will result in a complete left **homonymous hemianopia**. However, most optic tract lesions are partial, and because corresponding fibres from the nasal and retinal fields are not so close together in the tract, the homonymous hemianopia produced is incongruous (i.e. the hemi-field defect from the right eye is not an identical shape to that of the left) (4 on figure).

5 Meyer's loop

A lesion of the optic radiation in the temporal lobe will affect Meyer's loop, which contains fibres representing the inferior quadrant of the ipsilateral temporal retina, and the contralateral nasal retina. This results in a **superior homonymous quadrantanopia**, sometimes referred to as a 'pie in the sky' defect (5 on figure).

6 Parietal lobe

A lesion in the parietal lobe may affect the fibres from the superior quadrants of the ipsilateral temporal and contralateral nasal retina, giving rise to an **inferior homonymous quadrantanopia** or a homonymous hemianopia denser below than above (6 on figure).

7,8 Optic radiation to occipital cortex

Any unilateral lesion affecting the more anterior portion of the occipital cortex will give rise to a homonymous hemianopia. Because of the close proximity of the cells representing the corresponding retinal points, the hemianopia will be **congruous** (7 on figure), unlike the incongruous hemianopia seen with an optic tract lesion (the more posterior the lesion, the more congruous the field defect). Because the macula has a large representation in the occipital cortex, and a dual blood supply, the central 5° of vision is maintained in an anterior cortical lesion—**macular sparing** (8 on figure).

9 Macular fibres at occipital cortex

A posterior lesion affecting one side of the occipital cortex will result in a **homonymous hemianopic scotomatous** field defect (9 on figure).

KEY POINTS

• Bitemporal hemianopia indicates a chiasmal lesion—most commonly a pituitary tumour.
• Left homonymous hemianopia indicates a right cortical brain lesion.
• Altitudinal field defect is typical of anterior ischaemic optic neuropathy.

Appendix: Red eye

Signs and symptoms of different causes of a red eye

Signs and Symptoms	Conjunctivitis	Subconjunctival haemorrhage	Corneal abrasion	Allergy	Iritis	Acute glaucoma	Corneal ulcer
History	Family/ friend	Trauma, hypertension	Injury	Hay fever, asthma, eczema	Nil or other inflammatory disease	Change of lighting	Contact lens, injury
Sensation	Grittiness	None, mild irritation	Pain, photophobia	Itching	Pain, photophobia	Pain, photophobia, nausea	Pain, photophobia
Vision	Normal	Normal	Decreased (if central)	Normal	Decreased	Decreased	Decreased
Discharge	Purulent/clear	None	Tearing	Mucus	Tearing	Tearing	Tearing and mucopurulent
Pupillary light reflex	Brisk	Brisk	Brisk	Brisk	Sluggish	Mid-dilated and fixed	May be sluggish
Conjunctival injection	Diffuse, tarsal area	Localized, bright red	Diffuse	Diffuse, tarsal area	Circumcorneal	Diffuse	Circumcorneal
Corneal appearance	Clear	Clear	Stains with fluorescein	Clear	Keratic precipitates	Cloudy cornea	Stains with fluorescein
Intraocular pressure	Normal	Normal	Normal	Normal	Normal or elevated	Markedly elevated	Normal or elevated
Basic management	Hygiene, may require topical antibiotics	Reassurance, check blood pressure	Padding, topical antibiotics	Topical antihistamine	Ophthalmic referral	Ophthalmic referral	Ophthalmic referral

Index

Note: page numbers in *italics* refer to figures, those in **bold** refer to tables.